# PSEUDO MEDICINE

# PSEUDOMEDICINE

Arguing against the medicalization of the mundane

Brian Pollo

Manila, Philippines

*For Salcedo Hall*

## Contents

# Part 0: Motivations

This book began in a coffee shop conversation that left me unsettled. A friend, articulate and accomplished, described with genuine distress her inability to focus on tedious administrative tasks at work. She spoke of feeling overwhelmed by sensory input in crowded spaces, of needing solitude to recharge after social interaction, of procrastinating on projects until deadline pressure forced completion. Then she said, almost apologetically, "I think I might have undiagnosed ADHD and autism. Everything I read about it just clicks."

Naturally, my immediate internal response was reflexive dismissal. She held an advanced degree. She had maintained steady employment for years. Her relationships appeared stable and fulfilling. She managed the complex logistics of adult life competently. By any clinical definition, she exhibited no functional impairment. The diagnostic labels she tentatively claimed seemed absurdly misapplied.

As I listened further, it emerged that beneath the diagnostic language lay genuine struggles that mattered to her lived experience. The administrative tasks she "couldn't focus on" caused her real anxiety, even if she ultimately completed them. The sensory overwhelm in crowds was not merely preference but something that felt, at least to her, qualitatively different from ordinary social fatigue. The procrastination pattern, while not preventing her from meeting deadlines, carried psychological costs she experienced as substantial.

What struck me most was the relief in her voice when she described discovering online communities discussing these experiences through diagnostic frameworks. She had found language, however imperfect, for patterns she had struggled to articulate. She had found others who shared similar experiences, who validated that her difficulties were real rather than character defects. The diagnostic labels, regardless of their clinical accuracy, were performing some other psychological function.

This conversation repeated itself, with variations, dozens of times over the subsequent months. Intelligent, functional people describing themselves as having ADHD, autism, anxiety, or depression based not on clinical assessment but on identification with symptom descriptions encountered online. Each time, my initial response was the same irritation at what seemed like trivialization of serious conditions, appropriation of clinical language for subclinical experiences, and participation in a cultural trend that was degrading the meaning of psychiatric diagnosis.

Yet each time, these were not people malingering for advantage or seeking attention. They were people struggling with aspects of their psychology or temperament that caused them genuine distress, searching for frameworks to understand and communicate their experiences, and finding the available non-clinical vocabulary inadequate to the task.

The tension crystallized: they were using diagnostic language incorrectly in ways that threatened the integrity of clinical categories, but they were doing so in service of legitimate needs that our culture has failed to address through other means. Both things were true simultaneously. The question was not whether to validate their experiences or preserve diagnostic rigor, but how to do both.

This book emerged from my reflection on that question. It represents an attempt to articulate why diagnostic expansion threatens genuine harm to severely impaired individuals who depend on clinical categories functioning properly, while simultaneously acknowledging the psychological and social needs that drive subclinical individuals toward diagnostic self-identification. The argument I develop attempts a defense of diagnostic boundaries, but I hope it proceeds with empathy for those whose search for validation and community has led them to cross those boundaries.

The stakes are not abstract. I have worked with individuals whose ADHD is so severe they cannot maintain employment despite normal intelligence, whose executive dysfunction produces cascading life failures despite desperate efforts at compensation. I have known autistic individuals who cannot navigate basic social interaction, who find the sensory environment so overwhelming that independent living becomes impossible, whose families struggle daily with profound caregiving demands. These individuals need psychiatric diagnosis to function as precise instruments identifying who requires intensive intervention. When those instruments become dulled through over-application to mild presentations, the severely impaired pay the price.

Yet I have also watched my friend struggle with aspects of her temperament and personality that cause her genuine difficulty, searching for frameworks that validate her experience without pathologizing her. I understand why the language of neurodivergence appeals: it offers explanation without moral judgment, community without stigma, and recognition that struggles are real even when they do not constitute clinical disorders.

The central argument of this book is that we can honor both imperatives, but only through conceptual discipline. Clinical diagnoses must be reserved for presentations meeting clear functional impairment criteria. Simultaneously, we must develop richer non-pathological vocabulary for discussing the full range of human psychological variation, acknowledging that traits exist on continua and can create challenges without reaching pathological thresholds.

This requires rejecting the notion (widely accepted in popular discourse) that validation of psychosocial struggles requires diagnostic labels. It does not. Someone can struggle genuinely with attention, organization, sensory processing, or social interaction without having ADHD, autism, or indeed, any disorder. Their struggles deserve recognition, support, and accommodation where appropriate, but recognition need not take the form of medical diagnosis when the criteria for medical diagnosis are not met.

The book's structure reflects this dual concern. The early chapters build a case against diagnostic expansion, documenting how it violates statistical principles, eliminates predictive validity, breaches conceptual parsimony, and harms the severely impaired through resource diversion and trivialization. The later chapters engage with the arguments for diagnostic expansion, particularly the therapeutic and anti-stigma rationales, acknowledging their identification of real needs while demonstrating why those needs cannot justify epistemic corruption.

Throughout, I have tried to remember my friend's voice describing her struggles with genuine distress, even as I argue she should not claim diagnoses she does not meet criteria for. The tension between compassion for individual experience and commitment to collective systems of meaning runs through every chapter. I believe that tension is ultimately resolvable, but only if we are willing to do the difficult cultural and linguistic work of developing frameworks for validation that do not depend on medical pathologization.

The title invokes "overmedicalization," but the deeper problem is something stranger: the appropriation of medical language for non-medical purposes. When someone describes mild distractibility as ADHD or preference for routine as autism, they are not seeking medicalization in the traditional sense of wanting medical treatment for their condition. Often they actively resist medical framing, preferring neurodiversity language that celebrates difference rather than pathologizing it. Yet they retain the diagnostic terminology, which derives its cultural power from its medical origins. This creates a hybrid discourse that uses clinical language while rejecting clinical standards, appropriating medical authority while abandoning medical rigor.

In this work, I argue that this discourse is untenable. Either diagnostic categories remain medical constructs governed by empirical criteria, or they become identity labels self-determined through personal identification. I hold that they cannot coherently be both. The consequences of that choice matter enormously for the individuals with genuine disabilities who depend on diagnostic systems functioning as intended.

My hope is that readers will come away with two convictions that might initially seem contradictory: first, that diagnostic boundaries must be maintained rigorously to protect the severely impaired; second, that the impulse driving people toward diagnostic self-identification reflects legitimate needs our culture must address through other means. The synthesis of these convictions requires creating cultural space for discussing psychological variation with nuance and compassion while preserving clinical categories for genuine pathology.

If I succeed with this book, it will help some readers recognize that the struggles they have been framing through diagnostic language might be better understood and addressed through different frameworks. It will equip others to advocate for diagnostic rigor while remaining empathetic to the needs that drive diagnostic expansion. Most importantly, it will contribute to protecting the conceptual infrastructure that individuals with severe impairments need to access care and accommodation.

The conversation in that coffee shop continues to haunt me. I failed, initially, to respond with sufficient empathy to my friend's search for understanding and validation. I hope this book represents a more adequate response: one that takes her struggles seriously while insisting that clinical language has specific meanings that must be preserved for those whose struggles reach different thresholds of severity. We can validate her experience and protect diagnostic clarity. We can offer her community and language without pathologizing her temperament. But only if we are willing to reject the premise that all recognition must flow through medical diagnosis.

That rejection, and the conceptual honesty it requires, is what this book ultimately advocates.

# Part 1: Erosion of Specificity

## 1.1. Continuum Fallacy and Symptomatic Bleed

The construction of psychiatric categories rests upon a mathematical substrate that pop psychology systematically misapprehends. Consider the operational reality of attention-deficit/hyperactivity disorder (ADHD) diagnosis. The disorder manifests through measurable deficits in executive function—specifically, working memory capacity, inhibitory control, and cognitive flexibility. These are not metaphysical essences but quantifiable neuropsychological parameters that distribute continuously across human populations.

Empirical studies employing continuous performance tests (CPTs) reveal that response inhibition errors and reaction time variability form normal distributions in the general population. The landmark Multimodal Treatment Study of Children with ADHD (MTA), which tracked 579 children across multiple sites, demonstrated that inattention and hyperactivity-impulsivity scores on the Swanson, Nollen, and Pelham (SNAP-IV) rating scale follow

Gaussian distributions with no natural inflection points separating "disordered" from "typical" populations. Russell Barkley's comprehensive neuropsychological batteries similarly show that deficits in behavioral inhibition—the core construct he identifies as central to ADHD—exist along a continuum with no categorical boundary.

The diagnostic threshold established by the DSM-5 requires functional impairment in two or more settings and the presence of symptoms before age twelve. Statistically, this corresponds approximately to individuals performing beyond two standard deviations (2σ) from the population mean on validated measures of executive dysfunction. At this threshold, we encounter approximately 2.3% of the population in the tail of a normal distribution—a figure remarkably consistent with rigorous epidemiological estimates of ADHD prevalence using strict diagnostic criteria, as reported in Polanczyk et al.'s 2007 meta-analysis of worldwide prevalence studies, which converged on 5.29% when accounting for methodological variance but dropped substantially when applying stringent impairment criteria.

The neurobiological substrate reinforces this dimensional view. Positron emission tomography (PET) studies by Nora Volkow and colleagues at the National Institute of Mental Health demonstrate that dopamine transporter (DAT) density in the striatum—

specifically the binding potential of [$^{11}$C]cocaine to DAT—correlates dimensionally with attention scores. Individuals diagnosed with ADHD show elevated DAT density, resulting in excessive dopamine reuptake and reduced synaptic availability. However, this elevation itself exists on a continuum; there is no discrete neurochemical cliff that separates clinical from subclinical presentations.

Digital discourse has systematically eroded these statistical boundaries through a process of semantic drift and threshold collapse. On platforms such as TikTok and Instagram, content tagged #ADHD has accumulated over 30 billion views as of 2024. Qualitative analysis of this content reveals a consistent pattern: common human experiences of task avoidance, boredom during unstimulating activities, or preference for novelty are reframed as pathognomonic signs of neurological disorder.

Consider a representative example: a video with 4.2 million views presents "forgetting why you entered a room" as an ADHD symptom. Yet this phenomenon—environmental context-dependent memory failure—is a universal feature of human cognition documented extensively by Godden and Baddeley's classic 1975 study on state-dependent retrieval. The mechanism involves the encoding specificity principle: memory retrieval is optimized when contextual cues at encoding match those at retrieval. Room transitions disrupt this match for all humans, not selectively for those with executive dysfunction.

The statistical consequence is catastrophic. If we accept the pop psychology framing—where any instance of distractibility, procrastination, hyperfocus during interesting activities, or sensory preference constitutes evidence of ADHD—the diagnostic category expands to encompass the central 68% of the population (within 1σ), or even the central 95% (within 2σ), depending on how liberally symptoms are interpreted. This renders the diagnosis vacuously true through a process logicians call concept inflation: when a term becomes applicable to nearly all members of a domain, it loses definitional utility.

The philosopher Karl Popper established that scientific claims must possess falsifiability—the logical possibility of disconfirmation. A diagnosis that applies to 70% of the population based on everyday experiences fails this criterion. It becomes an unfalsifiable tautology: if virtually everyone exhibits the "symptoms," the construct no longer distinguishes a pathological minority from typical variation.

Autism spectrum disorder (ASD) diagnosis has suffered parallel distortion. The clinical reality of autism involves profound impairments in social communication, often accompanied by restricted, repetitive behaviors that cause significant functional limitations. The Social Responsiveness Scale (SRS-2), a quantitative measure validated by John Constantino and colleagues, reveals that social communication abilities distribute normally in the population. Clinical autism diagnoses correspond to scores approximately 2.5σ to 3σ from the mean—individuals whose social cognitive deficits are severe enough to require substantial support.

The diagnostic gold standards (*i.e.,* the Autism Diagnostic Observation Schedule (ADOS-2) and Autism Diagnostic Interview-Revised (ADI-R)) employ algorithmic cutoffs calibrated against these statistical thresholds. These instruments assess specific behaviors such as lack of social-emotional reciprocity, absent or abnormal eye contact, failure to develop peer relationships, and marked impairment in nonverbal communication. Critically, these must be present early in development and cause clinically significant impairment.

Pop psychology has focused particularly on sensory processing differences. Content claiming "if you hate certain textures, you might be autistic" has proliferated extensively. Yet sensory processing sensitivity exists dimensionally in the general population. Elaine Aron's research on the sensory processing sensitivity trait demonstrates that approximately 15-20% of the population exhibits heightened sensory awareness—a temperamental characteristic distributed normally and distinct from autism. The preference for soft versus scratchy fabrics, sensitivity to fluorescent lighting, or discomfort with loud environments are common human variations in sensory threshold, mediated by individual differences in sensory gating mechanisms at the level of the thalamic reticular nucleus.

Neuroscientific evidence supports this dimensional view. Functional MRI studies by Marco Iacoboni examining mirror neuron system (MNS) activity—particularly in the inferior frontal gyrus and inferior parietal lobule—show that while individuals with autism often exhibit reduced MNS activation during social observation tasks, this reduction exists on a continuum. There is no discrete neurobiological boundary; rather, a smooth gradient of mirror neuron responsivity correlates with social cognitive ability across the population.

The dimensional nature of these conditions reflects their underlying biology. ADHD and autism are polygenic conditions influenced by hundreds of common genetic variants, each of small effect. The 2023 genome-wide association study (GWAS) by Demontis et al., analyzing 38,691 individuals with ADHD, identified twelve genome-wide significant loci but demonstrated that the genetic architecture is massively polygenic. The SNP-based heritability ($h^2$) is approximately 0.22, distributed across the genome without major effect genes. This creates a liability threshold model: individuals inherit varying numbers of risk alleles, producing a continuous distribution of genetic loading. Only those exceeding a threshold—combining high genetic risk with environmental factors—manifest clinically significant impairment.

The dopaminergic hypothesis of ADHD illustrates this dimensional mechanism. The genes most consistently associated with ADHD—DAT1 (SLC6A3), DRD4, DRD5—modulate dopamine signaling efficiency. The 10-repeat allele of the DAT1 variable number tandem repeat (VNTR) polymorphism produces higher dopamine transporter expression, increasing dopamine clearance from the synapse. However, this allele exists in approximately 70% of the population with varying copy numbers and expression levels. The clinical phenotype emerges from cumulative effects across multiple genes in this pathway, moderated by environmental factors such as prenatal nicotine exposure or early childhood adversity.

Similarly, autism's genetic architecture involves synaptic genes (SHANK3, NLGN3, NLGN4), chromatin remodeling genes (CHD8), and genes regulating cortical development. The 2019 GWAS meta-analysis by Grove et al., examining 18,381 autism cases, revealed that common variation explains approximately 50% of autism liability, but this is distributed across thousands of loci. The continuous genetic liability translates into continuous variation in social cognitive capacity, with clinical autism representing the extreme tail.

The structure of psychiatric diagnosis specifies conditions under which intervention is warranted based on functional impairment. The DSM-5 explicitly requires that symptoms cause "clinically significant distress or impairment in social, occupational, or other important areas of functioning". This is not merely descriptive but normatively loaded: diagnosis implies the patient's condition reaches a threshold where medical intervention is justified and potentially obligatory from a healthcare ethics standpoint.

Pop psychology has inverted this framework. Rather than diagnosis emerging from demonstrated impairment, self-identification precedes and supplants clinical assessment. The phrase "self-diagnosed ADHD" has become commonplace, appearing in 847,000 TikTok videos as of late 2024. This represents a category error: diagnosis is not a speech act of self-declaration but the outcome of a systematic evaluative process comparing an individual's functioning against population norms using validated instruments.

The philosopher Ian Hacking's concept of "looping effects" illuminates this phenomenon. As psychiatric categories enter public discourse, they alter the subjective experience and self-understanding of individuals, who then reshape the category through their enactment of it. ADHD has undergone particularly aggressive looping: the pop culture version—characterized by quirky distractibility and creative thinking—bears minimal resemblance to the clinical reality of executive dysfunction severe enough to prevent completion of education, maintenance of employment, or management of basic life responsibilities.

This semantic drift has measurable consequences. Stephen Hinshaw's longitudinal studies following girls with ADHD into adulthood reveal that untreated clinical ADHD predicts substantially elevated rates of self-injury, suicide attempts, and serious accidents. The median annual income for adults with childhood ADHD is significantly lower than controls. These are not individuals who occasionally forget appointments or prefer stimulating activities—these are individuals whose executive dysfunction prevents them from executing long-term plans, maintaining relationships, or regulating emotional responses to frustration.

The logical error underlying pop psychology's diagnostic expansion is the confusion of necessary conditions with sufficient conditions. Consider the syllogistic structure:

**Premise 1:** All individuals with clinical ADHD experience distractibility.

**Premise 2:** I experience distractibility. **Conclusion:** Therefore, I have ADHD.

This commits the formal fallacy of affirming the consequent. Distractibility is a necessary condition for ADHD diagnosis (if ADHD, then distractibility) but not a sufficient condition (distractibility does not entail ADHD). The sufficient condition requires the conjunction of multiple symptoms at threshold severity plus demonstrated functional impairment across settings plus early onset plus exclusion of alternative explanations.

Epidemiological data starkly illustrate this distinction. Surveys of the general population reveal that approximately 60-70% of adults report experiencing significant difficulty maintaining attention on unstimulating tasks. However, rigorous epidemiological studies using structured clinical in1erviews—such as the National Comorbidity Survey Replication, which employed the World Health Organization's Composite International Diagnostic Interview (CIDI)—find adult ADHD prevalence of 4.4%. The 15-fold discrepancy between symptom endorsement and clinical diagnosis reflects the distance between necessary and sufficient conditions.

The continuum fallacy represents more than semantic imprecision—it constitutes epistemic violence against clinical reality. When pop psychology collapses distributional boundaries, treating common human variation as pathology, it simultaneously trivializes genuine disorder and pathologizes normalcy. The person with mild executive inefficiency who self-identifies with ADHD based on TikTok videos appropriates a diagnosis while potentially obscuring the experience of individuals like those in Hinshaw's longitudinal cohort, whose lives are devastated by severe executive dysfunction.

The restoration of diagnostic validity requires reasserting statistical precision. Clinical diagnoses are not identity categories but probabilistic statements about an individual's position on a dimensional trait distribution relative to functional impairment thresholds. They are tools for identifying who requires intervention, not labels for expressing personality or explaining quotidian human struggles.

The neuroscientist Robert Sapolsky observes that human behavior exists at the intersection of multiple continuous distributions—genetic, developmental, neurochemical. Clinical categories are artificial constructs we impose on this continuity for pragmatic purposes. Their utility depends entirely on maintaining clear thresholds calibrated to genuine impairment. Pop psychology's erasure of these boundaries does not democratize diagnosis—it destroys it, leaving us unable to distinguish those who need help from those who simply need to be human.

## 1.2. Loss of Predictive Validity

A medical diagnosis serves as more than descriptive nomenclature. It functions as a predictive instrument, a compressed representation of probabilistic information about future trajectories. When a clinician assigns a diagnosis of major depressive disorder, this determination carries embedded predictions: without intervention, the patient faces elevated risk of suicide attempt, occupational disability, social withdrawal, and recurrent episodes. The diagnosis justifies specific therapeutic interventions because it predicts outcomes that those interventions can modify.

This predictive function grounds the scientific legitimacy of psychiatric nosology. Thomas Insel, former director of the National Institute of Mental Health, argued that psychiatric diagnoses must demonstrate predictive validity to warrant their existence as natural kinds. A valid diagnostic category should predict treatment response, longitudinal course, biological markers, and functional outcomes with greater accuracy than chance or than broader dimensional measures. Without such predictive power, a category becomes scientifically arbitrary, no matter how reliable its symptomatic criteria.

The Research Domain Criteria (RDoC) initiative, which Insel championed, emerged partly from concerns that DSM categories lacked adequate predictive validity. RDoC proposed organizing psychopathology around dimensional constructs like working memory capacity or reward sensitivity rather than categorical syndromes. The debate between categorical and dimensional approaches hinges precisely on which framework better predicts what matters: suffering, disability, treatment response, and life trajectory.

Pop psychology has inadvertently conducted a massive uncontrolled experiment testing the predictive validity of diluted diagnostic categories. By expanding diagnostic boundaries to include subclinical presentations, it has created two populations bearing the same label: those meeting rigorous clinical criteria with demonstrated functional impairment, and those self-identifying based on mild trait elevation or relatable symptom descriptions. Comparing outcomes between these groups reveals whether the diagnosis retains meaning when severed from impairment thresholds.

The Berkeley Girls with ADHD Longitudinal Study, directed by Stephen Hinshaw beginning in 1997, provides exceptional data on life trajectories for rigorously diagnosed ADHD. The study recruited 140 girls meeting full DSM-IV criteria for ADHD with documented impairment, matched against 88 comparison girls. Diagnosis required comprehensive assessment including structured diagnostic interviews, teacher and parent rating scales, and direct observation during standardized tasks. Critically, impairment criteria were strictly enforced: participants demonstrated significant academic underperformance relative to intellectual ability, peer relationship difficulties, or family conflict directly attributable to ADHD symptoms.

The 16-year follow-up data, published by Hinshaw and Blachman in 2018, document stark outcomes. By young adulthood, 51% of girls with childhood ADHD had attempted suicide, compared to 13% of controls. Self-injury rates reached 56% versus 22%. Educational attainment lagged substantially: only 29% of the ADHD group completed a four-year college degree, compared to 68% of controls, despite no differences in measured intelligence at baseline. Rates of teenage pregnancy were nearly four times higher in the ADHD group.

These outcomes manifest through identifiable mechanisms. Executive function deficits produce academic underperformance not through lack of intelligence but through inability to organize long-term projects, inhibit distracting behaviors during study, or maintain goal-directed effort when rewards are delayed. Emotional dysregulation, particularly difficulty modulating frustration responses, precipitates conflicts with peers, romantic partners, and employers. Impulsivity predicts risky sexual behavior, substance experimentation, and reckless driving. The diagnosis predicts these outcomes precisely because it identifies genuine neurocognitive vulnerabilities.

Rachel Klein's longitudinal study of boys with ADHD, initiated in the 1970s and following participants for over three decades, reveals parallel trajectories. Men diagnosed with ADHD in childhood showed substantially elevated rates of substance use disorders, criminal justice involvement, and unemployment in adulthood. The hazard ratio for developing antisocial personality disorder was 4.5 for the ADHD group relative to controls. Notably, these elevated risks persisted even after controlling for childhood conduct problems, suggesting ADHD-specific mechanisms related to poor impulse control and deficient consideration of future consequences.

Contrast these trajectories with outcomes for individuals scoring in the subclinical range on ADHD symptom measures. Margaret Sibley's work examining young adults with subthreshold ADHD symptoms provides instructive data. Her studies identify individuals scoring between 1.0 and 1.5 standard deviations above the mean on continuous ADHD rating scales but not meeting full diagnostic criteria, particularly the functional impairment requirement. These individuals report attention difficulties and organizational challenges but maintain adequate academic performance, stable employment, and functional relationships.

Longitudinal follow-up of this subthreshold group reveals outcomes nearly identical to the general population. College completion rates, employment stability, relationship quality, and psychological well-being at five-year follow-up do not differ significantly from matched controls with minimal ADHD symptoms. The mild elevation in trait scores does not predict meaningful life difficulties. This demonstrates empirically that symptomatic threshold matters: the diagnosis predicts adverse outcomes only when symptoms reach sufficient severity to cause functional impairment.

The mechanism underlying this divergence relates to compensatory capacity. Individuals with mild attentional inefficiencies can deploy compensatory strategies: external scaffolding through calendars and reminders, selection into careers matching their attentional profile, or simply exerting greater conscious effort during demanding tasks. Clinical ADHD exceeds the threshold where compensation remains effective. The person cannot maintain employment even with external supports, cannot complete a college semester even with accommodations, cannot sustain a relationship even with a patient partner. Impairment criteria identify this threshold where inherent capacity falls below environmental demands.

Major depressive disorder provides another domain where predictive validity hinges on severity thresholds. The Patient Health Questionnaire (PHQ-9), developed by Kurt Kroenke and colleagues, quantifies depressive symptoms on a continuous scale from 0 to 27. A score of 10 or above suggests moderate depression warranting treatment. However, the instrument's real utility lies in its predictive validity at different thresholds.

Louzon et al.'s 2016 analysis of over 84,000 PHQ-9 administrations in military veterans examined suicide prediction across the severity spectrum. For patients scoring 5 to 9 (mild depression), suicide attempt rate over the subsequent year was 0.8%, only marginally elevated above the general veteran population baseline of 0.6%. For those scoring 20 or above (severe depression), the rate jumped to 4.2%, a sevenfold increase. The diagnosis of major depressive disorder predicts suicide risk specifically because diagnostic criteria select patients at this elevated-risk threshold.

The Beck Depression Inventory (BDI), developed by Aaron Beck in 1961, demonstrates similar threshold effects for functional outcomes. Longitudinal studies tracking individuals across the BDI severity spectrum show that those in the minimal range (0-13) maintain normal occupational functioning and social engagement. Those crossing into the moderate range (20-28) begin showing work productivity declines, but most remain employed. Severe depression (29-63) predicts occupational disability in over 60% of cases within six months. The clinical diagnosis aims to identify individuals in this severe range where intervention becomes necessary to prevent catastrophic functional decline.

Pop psychology's expansion of depression discourse to encompass transient sadness, disappointment, or stress responses eliminates this predictive utility. If someone describes feeling "depressed" after a romantic breakup or job rejection, this self-label provides no information about suicide risk, functional capacity, or need for intervention. The term has been severed from the clinical construct it originally denoted.

Predictive validity extends to treatment response. Clinical diagnoses should predict which patients will benefit from specific interventions. The degradation of diagnostic boundaries obscures these predictions, potentially exposing individuals without genuine pathology to unnecessary treatments while generating skepticism about interventions that benefit truly impaired patients.

The National Institute of Mental Health's Multimodal Treatment Study of Children with ADHD (MTA study) provides gold-standard evidence on treatment response. Children meeting rigorous ADHD diagnostic criteria, including documented school impairment and direct observation of inattention during cognitive testing, were randomized to medication management, behavioral therapy, combined treatment, or community care. Those receiving optimized stimulant medication (primarily methylphenidate) showed substantial symptom reduction: effect sizes of 0.8 to 1.0 on teacher-rated attention and hyperactivity, with corresponding improvements in academic productivity and peer relationships.

Crucially, these robust medication responses depend on accurate diagnosis. Studies administering stimulants to children with elevated ADHD symptom scores but no functional impairment show minimal benefit. The medication improves focus and productivity even in healthy controls, as demonstrated by Martha Farah's studies of cognitive enhancement in college students, but this represents performance enhancement in already-functional individuals rather than restoration of impaired function. The clinical diagnosis predicts a qualitatively different response: movement from dysfunctional to functional, not from functional to enhanced.

Similar patterns emerge in depression treatment. The STAR*D trial, the largest investigation of antidepressant effectiveness ever conducted, enrolled over 4,000 patients with major depressive disorder diagnosed using structured clinical interviews requiring both sufficient symptom number and functional impairment. Patients meeting these criteria showed 47% remission rates with initial SSRI treatment. By contrast, studies administering SSRIs to individuals with elevated depression symptom scores but minimal functional impairment show remission rates barely exceeding placebo, typically 35% for medication versus 30% for placebo.

Jay Fournier's meta-analysis published in JAMA examined antidepressant efficacy across the depression severity spectrum. For patients with Hamilton Depression Rating Scale scores below 23 (moderate severity), antidepressants provided minimal benefit over placebo: effect size approximately 0.20. Only at scores above 28 (severe depression) did benefit become clinically meaningful: effect size 0.50. This threshold corresponds closely to DSM functional impairment criteria. The clinical diagnosis predicts treatment response precisely because it identifies patients whose pathology reaches the threshold where pharmacological intervention affects outcomes.

Diagnostic validity manifests clearly in predictions about functional capacity. The National Comorbidity Survey Replication, conducted by Ronald Kessler and colleagues, assessed over 9,000 adults using structured diagnostic interviews for DSM-IV disorders. The study examined work productivity and unemployment across different levels of psychopathology.

Adults meeting full criteria for ADHD with impairment showed unemployment rates of 18%, compared to 7% in the general population. Among those employed, they missed an average of 9.5 additional workdays annually due to ADHD-related difficulties and experienced significant productivity loss on an additional 22 days. By contrast, adults with elevated ADHD symptom scores but no functional impairment showed unemployment rates of 8% and missed only 1.2 additional workdays, statistically indistinguishable from the general population.

The predictive gap appears even more starkly in autism spectrum disorder. Catherine Lord's longitudinal studies tracking children diagnosed with autism using gold-standard ADOS assessments reveal that those meeting diagnostic cutoffs in childhood show substantially restricted adult outcomes. At age 30, only 15% were competitively employed, and 65% still lived with parents or in supervised settings. These individuals had been diagnosed based not merely on social communication differences but on pervasive impairments preventing independent navigation of social demands.

Contrast this with outcomes for individuals with subclinical autistic traits measured by Simon Baron-Cohen's Autism Spectrum Quotient (AQ). Adults scoring in the elevated range (26-32 out of 50) but not meeting diagnostic criteria show employment rates and residential independence nearly identical to the general population. Their mild social cognitive differences do not predict functional disability. Some even show occupational advantages in fields requiring systematic thinking and attention to detail, such as engineering or computer programming.

The proliferation of self-diagnosis directly tests whether symptomatic identification alone, absent clinical confirmation of impairment, retains predictive validity. Surveys on social media platforms reveal that millions of young adults self-identify as having ADHD or autism based on relatability to content describing symptoms. This creates an unintentional natural experiment: do self-identified cases show the adverse outcomes predicted by clinical diagnosis?

Available evidence suggests they do not. Anastasia Hronis's 2022 study examined Australian young adults who self-identified as having ADHD based on social media content but had never pursued clinical assessment. The study tracked this group alongside clinically diagnosed individuals and matched controls over 18 months. The self-identified group showed no elevation in objective functional impairment measures: academic grades, employment stability, and relationship quality all fell within normal ranges. Subjective distress was elevated, but this appeared attributable to anxiety about potentially having ADHD rather than actual ADHD-related functional impairment.

This outcome divergence demonstrates that the self-applied label lacks predictive validity. When diagnostic expansion occurs through lowered thresholds and elimination of impairment criteria, the resulting category fails to predict the outcomes that justify clinical attention and intervention. A diagnosis that applies equally to someone completing graduate school while maintaining a career and healthy relationships, and to someone who has dropped out of high school and cannot maintain employment, has lost its ability to compress useful information about likely trajectories.

From a philosophical standpoint, the loss of predictive validity represents the dissolution of construct validity. A scientific construct must carve nature at its joints, identifying a coherent pattern of co-occurring features with shared etiology. When diagnostic boundaries expand to include qualitatively different presentations, the construct becomes incoherent.

Paul Meehl's concept of taxometrics provides a framework for understanding this dissolution. Meehl argued that valid psychiatric categories should demonstrate taxonic structure: a latent categorical distinction between affected and unaffected individuals, even if measured dimensionally. Statistical techniques can detect this structure by examining patterns of covariation among symptoms. If symptoms covary in a manner suggesting two distinct distributions (affected versus unaffected), a taxon exists. If symptoms simply correlate dimensionally without evidence of latent classes, the category is arbitrary.

Applying taxometric analysis to ADHD symptoms produces mixed results that illuminate the validity problem. Studies examining samples recruited from clinics serving highly impaired children detect taxonic structure: a distinct ADHD class separable from typical variation. However, studies using community samples with broader symptom ranges find dimensional structure without clear taxa. This suggests that clinical ADHD represents a coherent taxon, but only when impairment criteria sharply bound the category. As diagnostic boundaries blur through pop psychology's inclusiveness, the taxonic structure disappears into continuous variation.

The base rate inflation inherent in pop psychology's diagnostic expansion mathematically guarantees loss of predictive validity. Bayes' theorem demonstrates that as the prevalence of a condition increases in a population, the positive predictive value of any diagnostic indicator decreases. If genuine ADHD affects 5% of the population and a test correctly identifies 90% of cases with 10% false positives, the positive predictive value is 83%. If we expand the definition such that 40% of the population qualifies, the same test now has a positive predictive value of only 36%. The diagnosis becomes minimally informative.

The loss of predictive validity carries practical consequences beyond philosophical interest. Clinicians rely on diagnosis to guide treatment decisions. If half the patients diagnosed with ADHD show no functional impairment and no elevated risk of adverse outcomes, the diagnosis provides no guidance about who requires intervention. Treatment becomes arbitrary, applied based on subjective distress or patient demand rather than predicted benefit.

Research suffers parallel contamination. Studies enrolling participants based on broadened diagnostic criteria include heterogeneous samples combining genuinely impaired individuals with those experiencing normal-range variation. This heterogeneity inflates variance, reduces statistical power, and obscures genuine effects. Biological studies searching for neural or genetic markers of ADHD find weak, inconsistent results partly because samples include individuals without the neurobiological vulnerabilities the research aims to identify.

The philosopher of science Carl Hempel argued that scientific concepts must demonstrate empirical adequacy: they must facilitate successful prediction and explanation in the domain they purport to describe. Psychiatric diagnoses, as scientific concepts, must meet this standard. When pop psychology dilutes diagnostic categories by eliminating impairment criteria and expanding symptomatic thresholds, the resulting concepts fail Hempel's test. They no longer predict outcomes with sufficient accuracy to justify their use in scientific or clinical contexts.

The restoration of predictive validity requires re-establishing clear boundaries grounded in functional impairment. Diagnosis should identify individuals whose difficulties exceed what compensatory strategies can ameliorate, whose trajectories predict adverse outcomes absent intervention, and whose condition responds meaningfully to treatment. Absent these features, we possess not a diagnosis but merely a descriptive label for common human variation, stripped of the scientific and clinical utility that justifies diagnostic practice.

# Part 2: Exploring Backing

## 2.1. Conceptual Parsimony

William of Ockham never imagined his razor would need sharpening against the diagnostic enthusiasm of twenty-first century internet discourse, yet the fourteenth-century Franciscan friar articulated a principle whose violation now threatens the coherence of psychiatric nosology. Ockham's parsimony principle holds that entities should not be multiplied beyond necessity, that explanatory frameworks should employ the minimum conceptual apparatus sufficient to account for observed phenomena. Applied to psychiatric classification, parsimony demands that clinical diagnostic categories be invoked only when ordinary psychological vocabulary proves insufficient to capture the nature and severity of human difficulties. The proliferation of clinical labels for subclinical experiences represents not an expansion of medical understanding but a violation of this fundamental epistemic principle, introducing conceptual redundancy that degrades rather than enhances our descriptive capacity.

The principle of parsimony operates not as mere aesthetic preference but as epistemic necessity. Scientific progress depends on the creation of new concepts when existing vocabulary cannot adequately capture novel phenomena or when new theoretical frameworks reveal previously unrecognized natural kinds. The introduction of the concept "oxygen" by Antoine Lavoisier was warranted because phlogiston theory could not adequately explain combustion and respiration patterns. The concept "electron" became necessary when electromagnetic phenomena demanded positing subatomic particles. These conceptual innovations satisfied parsimony because they explained phenomena that existing concepts could not accommodate. The question facing psychiatric nosology is whether clinical diagnostic labels applied to mild personality variations similarly satisfy this criterion or whether they merely rename phenomena already adequately described by ordinary language.

Consider the ordinary language available for describing variations in attentional capacity and organizational skill. English provides a rich vocabulary: distractible, absent-minded, disorganized, forgetful, scatterbrained, unfocused, careless, hasty, impulsive, restless, fidgety. These terms communicate effectively in daily discourse, conveying information about behavioral tendencies that interlocutors readily understand without invoking pathology. A person described as "disorganized" evokes a clear image: someone whose workspace is cluttered, who misplaces belongings, who may arrive late to appointments. This description suffices for most purposes, allowing others to adjust expectations and accommodate the person's tendencies without medical framing.

The question parsimony poses is stark: what explanatory or descriptive work does the label "ADHD" accomplish for someone whose difficulties this ordinary vocabulary already captures? If a person occasionally forgets appointments, sometimes procrastinates on tedious tasks, and prefers stimulating activities to boring ones, but maintains employment, completes educational programs, and navigates relationships successfully, what does the clinical diagnosis add to the simpler description "somewhat disorganized" or "easily bored"? The diagnostic label multiplies entities, introducing the apparatus of medical pathology, without explaining anything the ordinary language could not.

Parsimony becomes particularly compelling when we examine the historical trajectory of attention concepts in psychology. William James devoted substantial discussion to attention in his 1890 Principles of Psychology without invoking pathological categories. James described attention as inherently selective, noting that consciousness cannot simultaneously process all available stimuli and must continually choose focus objects. He recognized individual differences: some minds wander readily, others sustain focus effortlessly. Yet James required no disease category to explain these variations. The ordinary concepts of "strong will" versus "weak will," "disciplined mind" versus "vagrant mind" sufficed to capture the relevant distinctions.

The construction of ADHD as a diagnostic category occurred gradually through the twentieth century. George Still's 1902 lectures to the Royal College of Physicians described children with "defective moral control" and abnormal incapacity for sustained attention, but Still was describing children whose difficulties were so severe as to make them "impossible" in educational settings. Charles Bradley's 1937 discovery that amphetamine improved behavior in institutionalized children similarly involved profoundly impaired individuals. The diagnostic category that eventually crystallized as ADHD was calibrated to identify this extreme tail: children whose attentional and behavioral difficulties exceeded what teachers and parents could manage through ordinary disciplinary and educational approaches.

The conceptual violation occurs when this category, carefully constructed to identify extreme impairment, gets applied to individuals whose difficulties fall within the range ordinary language already describes. A child who daydreams during boring lectures but completes assignments successfully does not require a medical diagnosis. The ordinary concept "daydreamer" or "restless when bored" captures the relevant information without invoking neurobiological pathology. Applying the ADHD label to such a child multiplies entities unnecessarily, adding the entire conceptual apparatus of disorder, impairment, neurological dysfunction, and treatment need where simpler psychological concepts would suffice.

The philosopher Willard Van Orman Quine developed a sophisticated account of ontological commitment, arguing that our theories commit us to believing in the existence of whatever entities those theories quantify over. When we describe someone using ordinary psychological language ("Sarah is disorganized"), we commit to believing in Sarah and in the property of being disorganized, but not to any underlying disease entity. When we diagnose Sarah with ADHD, we commit to believing in ADHD as a natural kind, a real pathological entity that Sarah possesses. This ontological commitment carries substantial weight: it posits that something is wrong with Sarah at a biological level, that she suffers from a medical condition requiring potential pharmaceutical intervention.

Quine's criterion of ontological commitment applies directly to diagnostic parsimony. We should accept ontological commitments only when explanatory necessity demands them. If Sarah's disorganization can be adequately understood and responded to using ordinary psychological concepts, positing an underlying disease entity violates parsimony. We introduce an unnecessary ontological commitment, cluttering our conceptual scheme with entities that do no explanatory work beyond what simpler concepts already accomplish.

The neuroscience of attention provides instructive examples of where clinical categories do satisfy parsimony and where they do not. Michael Posner's influential model of attention distinguishes three anatomically separable networks: alerting (maintained by noradrenergic projections from the locus coeruleus), orienting (controlled by cholinergic input to posterior parietal cortex), and executive control (dependent on dopaminergic signaling in anterior cingulate cortex and prefrontal regions). Individual differences in the efficiency of these networks exist across the population, measured by reaction time paradigms like the Attention Network Test.

For most individuals, these differences in network efficiency remain within functional range. Someone with slightly less efficient executive attention may take longer to inhibit prepotent responses or switch between tasks but can compensate through conscious effort or external scaffolding. The ordinary concepts of "distractible" or "impulsive" adequately describe this person's attentional profile without invoking pathology. Clinical ADHD diagnosis becomes parsimonious only for individuals whose executive attention network efficiency falls so far below population norms that compensation fails: their performance on sustained attention tasks is so impaired that they cannot complete educational programs despite adequate intelligence, cannot maintain employment despite effort, cannot regulate behavior sufficiently to avoid repeated accidents or conflicts.

This threshold demarcates where ordinary psychological concepts prove insufficient and clinical categories become necessary. Below this threshold, parsimony demands we use ordinary language. Above this threshold, ordinary language fails to capture the qualitative difference between normal-range inefficiency and pathological impairment. The clinical diagnosis "ADHD" then does genuine conceptual work, marking a discontinuity that ordinary vocabulary cannot express.

The inflation of diagnostic categories through pop psychology systematically violates parsimony by applying clinical labels far below this threshold. When someone describes themselves as having ADHD because they sometimes forget where they placed their keys or feel restless during long meetings, they invoke clinical pathology where the ordinary concepts "forgetful" or "restless" would suffice. This multiplication of diagnostic entities beyond explanatory necessity degrades our conceptual ecology.

The degradation manifests in several ways. First, diagnostic inflation creates semantic confusion: the term "ADHD" now references a heterogeneous collection including both severely impaired individuals who cannot function independently and mildly disorganized individuals who forget occasional appointments. When someone mentions having ADHD, their interlocutor cannot determine whether this signals genuine disability requiring accommodation or simply personality quirks requiring minor adjustments. The diagnostic label has lost informational content through over-application.

Second, unnecessary diagnostic multiplication obscures the experiences of genuinely impaired individuals. When the same label applies to someone completing a graduate degree while working full-time and to someone who cannot finish high school despite normal intelligence, the label fails to communicate the severity and nature of impairment. The severely impaired individual's struggles become invisible, submerged in a heterogeneous category dominated numerically by the mildly affected.

Third, conceptual inflation generates spurious research findings. Studies enrolling participants based on broadened ADHD criteria include individuals whose attentional variations require no special explanation beyond normal range variation in executive function efficiency. Searches for biological markers then fail because the sample includes substantial numbers of people without pathological biology. The field suffers from conceptual noise: genuine signals become undetectable amid the static generated by category members who should never have been included.

The philosopher Nelson Goodman analyzed the logic of category formation, distinguishing natural kinds from arbitrary groupings. Natural kinds support induction: knowing an organism is a raven supports inferences about its other properties (blackness, intelligence, social behavior). Arbitrary groupings do not: knowing an object is "grue" (green if observed before time t, blue if observed after) supports no useful inferences. Goodman argued that projectible predicates, those supporting legitimate induction, correspond to genuine similarities in nature rather than arbitrary human classification.

Psychiatric diagnosis aspires to identify natural kinds in Goodman's sense. A valid diagnostic category should be projectible: knowing someone meets diagnostic criteria for major depressive disorder should support inferences about neurotransmitter function, treatment response, and longitudinal course. This projectibility depends on the category capturing a coherent natural phenomenon rather than an arbitrary collection of symptoms.

Parsimony connects directly to projectibility. When diagnostic categories expand to include heterogeneous presentations united only by surface symptomatic similarity, they lose projectibility. Knowing someone "has ADHD" under inflated criteria supports few reliable inferences because the category includes individuals with fundamentally different underlying conditions: some with genuine executive function impairments rooted in dopaminergic dysfunction, others with ordinary variation in temperamental traits like conscientiousness or openness to experience.

The Big Five personality model provides relevant psychological constructs that already capture much individual variation currently being reframed as pathological. Conscientiousness, one of the five factors, encompasses traits like organization, diligence, goal-directed planning, and impulse control. Individuals low in conscientiousness tend toward disorganization, procrastination, and distractibility. These tendencies are stable across adulthood, normally distributed in the population, and substantially heritable (roughly 40% of variance attributable to genetic factors). The ordinary concept "low in conscientiousness" describes this personality configuration without invoking pathology.

Research by Nigg et al. has examined the relationship between conscientiousness and ADHD symptoms. While clinical ADHD patients score very low on conscientiousness, substantial numbers of individuals in the general population also score low without meeting ADHD diagnostic criteria or experiencing functional impairment. These low-conscientiousness individuals are simply at one end of normal personality variation. Applying ADHD diagnosis to them multiplies entities unnecessarily: the personality construct already provides adequate description.

Similarly, the trait of sensory processing sensitivity, studied extensively by Elaine Aron, describes individuals who process sensory information more thoroughly, notice subtle environmental cues, and become overstimulated by intense sensory input. Approximately 20% of the population scores high on this temperamental trait. These individuals prefer quiet environments, find scratchy fabrics uncomfortable, and become overwhelmed in crowded spaces. Yet this trait describes normal variation in sensory threshold, likely related to individual differences in thalamic gating mechanisms and cortical excitability.

Pop psychology increasingly frames sensory sensitivity as evidence of autism or sensory processing disorder. Yet parsimony rebels: the ordinary concept "sensory sensitive" or "easily overstimulated" adequately describes these individuals. No additional clinical category is necessary unless sensitivity reaches levels preventing basic functioning. A person who prefers soft fabrics and dislikes loud restaurants has a personality preference, not a pathological condition. The clinical diagnosis becomes parsimonious only when sensory differences prevent the person from tolerating necessary environments like workplaces or schools despite accommodations.

The violation of parsimony carries ethical implications beyond conceptual efficiency. Medical diagnoses invoke a normative framework: they designate something as wrong requiring correction. This normative loading affects how individuals understand themselves and how others regard them. Viktor Frankl, Austrian psychiatrist and Holocaust survivor, argued that the medicalization of ordinary suffering robs individuals of meaning-making capacity. When we frame normal human struggles as symptoms of pathology, we encourage passive patient identity rather than active engagement with life's inherent difficulties.

Frankl's logotherapy emphasized that struggle and frustration are intrinsic to human existence, not pathological deviations requiring medical correction. A person who struggles with motivation, becomes easily distracted, or feels restless may simply be encountering the ordinary challenge of disciplining attention, a challenge that ancient Stoic philosophers like Marcus Aurelius and Epictetus described extensively without invoking disease categories. Marcus Aurelius's Meditations repeatedly addresses the difficulty of maintaining focus and resisting distraction, treating this as a universal human struggle requiring philosophical cultivation rather than a medical condition affecting some unfortunate individuals.

When we apply clinical diagnoses to individuals experiencing such ordinary struggles, we perform conceptual violence. We take an experience adequately understood through humanistic or philosophical frameworks and reframe it as neurobiological pathology. This reframing is not neutral: it changes how people understand their difficulties and what responses they consider appropriate. Someone who understands their distractibility as a personal challenge to overcome through habit cultivation approaches it differently than someone who understands it as symptomatic of a brain disorder requiring pharmaceutical management.

Physicians have obligations to sick patients but not to healthy individuals seeking enhancement. This ethical distinction depends on clear boundaries between pathology and normal variation. When diagnostic categories expand to include subclinical presentations, these boundaries blur, creating ethical confusion. Does a physician have an obligation to prescribe stimulants to a mildly distractible college student who self-diagnoses with ADHD? Under strict parsimony, the answer is no: the student's difficulties fall within normal range and can be addressed through non-medical means. But under inflated diagnostic criteria, the answer becomes unclear, and physicians face pressure to medicalize normal variation.

The proliferation of clinical labels for ordinary experiences represents a category error in the philosophical sense identified by Gilbert Ryle. Ryle argued that category mistakes occur when we treat concepts appropriate to one logical category as belonging to another. His famous example contrasts someone seeking the university after being shown colleges, libraries, and laboratories. The visitor commits a category error by treating "the university" as an additional entity parallel to its constituent parts rather than as the organizational structure those parts compose.

Pop psychology commits an analogous category error by treating clinical diagnoses as appropriate descriptors for experiences already adequately captured by ordinary psychological concepts. Someone who occasionally forgets appointments commits a category error by self-diagnosing with ADHD: they mistake a common human experience (occasional forgetfulness) for membership in a pathological category (executive dysfunction severe enough to prevent normal functioning). The clinical diagnosis belongs to a different logical category than the everyday experiences it is being applied to.

Wittgenstein's concept of family resemblance illuminates why diagnostic boundaries matter for parsimony. Wittgenstein argued that many concepts lack necessary and sufficient conditions for membership but instead group instances sharing overlapping similarities. His example of "game" includes activities as diverse as chess, football, and solitaire, united by no single defining feature but by networks of similarity. Clinical diagnoses function differently: they aim to identify natural kinds with defining features, not family resemblance concepts.

When diagnostic boundaries blur through pop psychology's inclusiveness, clinical categories devolve from natural kinds into family resemblance concepts. "ADHD" comes to reference a loose collection of experiences sharing only surface similarities: some severe executive dysfunction, some personality traits, some ordinary human forgetfulness, some anxiety manifesting as restlessness. The category loses coherence, becoming a family resemblance grouping that satisfies no useful scientific or clinical purpose.

Parsimony demands that we resist this devolution by maintaining clear boundaries calibrated to functional impairment. Clinical diagnoses should remain reserved for presentations that exceed what ordinary psychological vocabulary can adequately describe, presentations where the qualitative impairment demands medical conceptualization. For the vast majority of human variation in attention, organization, sensory sensitivity, and social communication, ordinary language suffices. We need no clinical labels for people who are simply forgetful, disorganized, sensitive, or shy. These ordinary concepts accomplish all necessary descriptive and explanatory work without multiplying diagnostic entities.

The restoration of conceptual parsimony requires physicians, researchers, and the broader culture to recognize when clinical categories are being invoked unnecessarily. Before applying a diagnostic label, we must ask: do existing non-clinical concepts already adequately describe this person's experiences? Can their difficulties be understood using ordinary psychological vocabulary? If so, parsimony forbids diagnostic application. Only when ordinary language proves insufficient to capture the severity and nature of impairment does the clinical diagnosis satisfy its epistemic burden and warrant its ontological commitment.

# 2.2. The Mandate of Resource Allocation

The emergency department at Massachusetts General Hospital operates under a formal triage protocol derived from battlefield medicine. When a patient arrives, nurses assess severity using standardized criteria, assigning one of five urgency levels. Level 1 indicates immediate life threat requiring instantaneous intervention. Level 5 designates minor complaints manageable with routine care. This stratification reflects an ethical imperative: when resources are finite and demand exceeds supply, allocation must prioritize those with greatest need. A system that treats chest pain and ingrown toenails identically would violate basic principles of medical ethics, allowing preventable deaths while expending resources on trivial complaints. Psychiatric diagnosis functions as a comparable triage system, identifying individuals whose cognitive or emotional difficulties reach thresholds justifying access to specialized interventions. The degradation of diagnostic boundaries through pop psychology does not merely introduce conceptual confusion. It actively harms severely impaired individuals by flooding support systems with people experiencing mild difficulties, creating artificial scarcity that prevents those with genuine disabilities from accessing necessary resources.

Distributive justice, as articulated by John Rawls in A Theory of Justice, demands that inequalities in resource distribution are justifiable only when they benefit the least advantaged members of society. Applied to disability services, this principle requires that accommodations and interventions flow preferentially to those most impaired, those whose capacity to function independently falls furthest below population norms. Educational accommodations like extended test time exist not to advantage students who might benefit marginally from additional minutes but to level the playing field for students whose disabilities would otherwise prevent them from demonstrating their knowledge despite adequate preparation. A student with severe dyslexia who reads at one-fifth normal speed requires extended time to access the same examination content as peers. A student who simply prefers working slowly does not face comparable disadvantage.

The formal structure of accommodation systems in American education reflects this prioritization through legal mechanisms. The Individuals with Disabilities Education Act, enacted in 1975 and reauthorized multiple times, guarantees students with disabilities access to Free Appropriate Public Education, including specialized instruction and related services. Section 504 of the Rehabilitation Act of 1973 prohibits discrimination against individuals with disabilities and mandates reasonable accommodations in educational settings. The Americans with Disabilities Act of 1990 extended these protections to employment and public accommodations. These laws share a common feature: they define disability through functional impairment criteria, requiring that conditions substantially limit one or more major life activities.

The legal framework instantiates an ethical commitment: society owes special obligations to individuals whose impairments prevent them from accessing opportunities available to others. A student whose ADHD is so severe that they cannot read a textbook chapter despite repeated attempts, whose mind wanders after every sentence despite desperate efforts to maintain focus, experiences a disability. This student cannot access education through normal means and requires accommodations to achieve educational access comparable to peers. Society's obligation to provide accommodations derives from this genuine inability, not from the student's mere preference for support or marginal difficulty with sustained attention.

Consider the resource constraints facing special education systems. The Los Angeles Unified School District, second largest in the United States, serves over

90,000 students with Individualized Education Programs as of 2023. These students receive specialized instruction from special education teachers, many of whom hold advanced credentials in working with specific disabilities. The student-to-teacher ratio in special education substantially exceeds that in general education to accommodate intensive individualized attention. Speech therapists, occupational therapists, behavioral specialists, and school psychologists provide additional services. The per-pupil expenditure for special education students averages roughly twice that of general education students, reflecting the intensive resources required.

These resources are finite. School districts employ a fixed number of special education teachers, maintain limited numbers of resource rooms, and budget predetermined amounts for evaluations and services. When the number of students requiring services increases, either resources must be stretched thinner across more students, wait times for evaluations must lengthen, or eligibility criteria must tighten. The system operates under resource constraints, making allocation decisions unavoidable.

The impact of diagnostic inflation on this system is mechanistically straightforward. When students with mild attentional variations begin seeking ADHD diagnoses and corresponding accommodations, they enter the queue for limited services. Psychologists conducting comprehensive evaluations spend hours administering cognitive batteries, attention tests, and processing speed measures to students whose difficulties may not reach impairment thresholds. Each evaluation consumes resources that could serve students with clear disabilities. When accommodations are granted to students with subclinical presentations, classroom teachers must track an increasing number of individualized plans, fragmenting their attention and reducing the intensive support available to students with severe disabilities.

Data from the National Center for Education Statistics document this expansion. Between 2000 and 2020, the percentage of students receiving services under IDEA's "other health impairment" category, which includes ADHD, increased from 1.1% to 1.6% of all public school students, a 45% relative increase. Concurrently, surveys of school psychologists reveal that wait times for comprehensive evaluations have lengthened substantially, with many districts reporting backlogs exceeding six months. Meanwhile, students with profound disabilities like intellectual disability or multiple disabilities have seen no corresponding increase in per-pupil resources. The expanding pool of accommodation recipients dilutes available resources.

The pharmaceutical dimension reveals even starker resource allocation failures. Stimulant medications constitute the first-line pharmacological treatment for ADHD. Methylphenidate, synthesized by Leandro Panizzon in 1944 and introduced commercially as Ritalin in 1954, works by blocking dopamine and norepinephrine reuptake, increasing catecholamine availability in the synaptic cleft. Amphetamine compounds, introduced even earlier, additionally promote neurotransmitter release through trace amine-associated receptor 1 activation and vesicular monoamine transporter 2 reversal. These mechanisms enhance prefrontal cortical function, improving working memory, response inhibition, and sustained attention in individuals with dopaminergic signaling deficits.

The therapeutic value of stimulants for genuinely impaired ADHD patients is substantial. The effect sizes in rigorously diagnosed populations range from 0.8 to 1.2, representing movement from the 21st percentile to the 50th percentile on attention measures. For children whose ADHD prevents them from remaining seated during class, completing assignments, or maintaining peer relationships, stimulant medication can represent the difference between educational failure and success. Russell Barkley documents cases where appropriately medicated children move from failing grades and disciplinary problems to grade-level performance and improved social functioning within months.

However, stimulant medications carry misuse potential and adverse effects. The mechanism that improves attention in ADHD patients also enhances cognitive performance in healthy individuals, as demonstrated by studies showing that amphetamine improves working memory and sustained attention even in adults with no attention difficulties. This creates a perverse incentive: individuals without genuine impairment seek diagnoses to access performance enhancement rather than disability remediation. Martha Farah's research at the University of Pennsylvania documented extensive stimulant use among college students for academic enhancement, with many obtaining prescriptions through strategic symptom reporting during evaluations.

The scope of this phenomenon is substantial. Surveys conducted by Sean McCabe at the University of Michigan reveal that between 5% and 35% of college students at competitive universities have used prescription stimulants non-medically, with rates highest at schools with rigorous academic demands. While some students obtain medications illicitly, others pursue formal diagnoses. The incentive structure is clear: a student facing intense academic competition who can obtain extended test time and stimulant medication gains competitive advantage.

The ethical violation operates at multiple levels. First, students obtaining accommodations and medications without genuine impairment consume resources that could benefit truly disabled students. Every prescription written for a mildly distractible student who performs adequately without medication represents methylphenidate that could have improved a severely impaired child's educational trajectory. Second, the proliferation of questionable diagnoses generates skepticism about accommodation legitimacy, making it harder for genuinely disabled students to access necessary supports without stigma. Third, manufacturing shortages of stimulant medications periodically create situations where demand exceeds supply, forcing difficult allocation decisions.

The Drug Enforcement Administration regulates stimulant production through aggregate production quotas calibrated to estimated medical need. In 2011, shortages of immediate-release amphetamine compounds left patients unable to fill prescriptions for months. While manufacturing issues contributed, the shortage reflected partly the explosive growth in stimulant prescribing, which increased roughly 300% between 1990 and 2010. When supply limitations emerge, pharmacies implement allocation protocols, but these rarely distinguish between patients with severe impairment requiring medication to function and those with mild symptoms seeking enhancement. The truly impaired often suffer alongside the questionably diagnosed.

Adult ADHD diagnosis presents an even more ethically fraught domain because accommodations and treatments in adult contexts directly affect competitive outcomes. The Law School Admission Test, Medical College Admission Test, and similar high-stakes examinations grant accommodations including extended time to examinees with documented disabilities. These accommodations are intended to ensure that examinations measure knowledge and reasoning rather than disability-related limitations. A student whose processing speed deficit causes them to read substantially slower than peers requires extended time to access the same test content others encounter.

However, extended time also benefits non-disabled examinees. Studies of standardized testing demonstrate that nearly all test-takers improve scores when given additional time, with gains typically in the range of 10-15 percentile points. This creates an obvious incentive: ambitious students seek ADHD diagnoses to gain competitive advantage in admissions processes. The psychologist Richard Atkinson, former president of the University of California system, has documented that students from affluent backgrounds obtain accommodation diagnoses at substantially higher rates than socioeconomically disadvantaged peers, likely reflecting differential access to evaluations and strategic gaming of diagnostic systems.

The result is an arms race where accommodation prevalence increases without corresponding increases in genuine disability prevalence. Collegeboard data indicate that the percentage of SAT examinees receiving accommodations increased from approximately 2% in 2000 to over 5% by 2020. Some of this increase likely reflects improved identification of previously underdiagnosed disabilities. However, substantial evidence suggests diagnostic threshold creep, with students experiencing mild difficulties increasingly obtaining diagnoses that previously would not have been rendered.

The economic incentives exacerbating this problem merit examination. Comprehensive neuropsychological evaluations cost between $2000 and $5000, creating a barrier for lower-income families but a manageable investment for affluent families seeking competitive advantage for their children. Private psychologists who conduct these evaluations face financial pressure to render diagnoses, as families dissatisfied with non-diagnostic conclusions may seek second opinions from more accommodating practitioners. The result is adverse selection: psychologists willing to apply diagnostic labels generously attract more referrals.

This dynamic creates severe inequity. Students from families with resources to purchase evaluations and navigate accommodation systems obtain support, while equally or more impaired students from low-income families go undiagnosed and unserved. Simultaneously, students with mild difficulties from affluent families obtain accommodations, consuming limited resources and contributing to the dilution of support available to the severely impaired. The system violates distributive justice principles by allowing wealth rather than need to determine resource access.

The harm to genuinely impaired individuals extends beyond resource dilution to stigma and delegitimization. When accommodations become common, perceived as advantages obtained through gaming rather than necessities for disability compensation, those with genuine disabilities face skepticism. Faculty members observing that 20% of students in a course request extended time may begin to doubt accommodation legitimacy, becoming less willing to provide flexible deadlines, alternative examination formats, or other supports. Students with genuine disabilities then face hostile environments where their needs are questioned.

Jennifer Crocker's research on stigma and legitimacy demonstrates this dynamic empirically. When members of a beneficiary group appear undeserving, stigma intensifies for all group members, including those with legitimate claims. In the disability context, the presence of students with questionable diagnoses obtaining accommodations generates suspicion that harms students with unambiguous disabilities. A student with severe dyslexia who struggles to read despite normal intelligence faces implicit accusations of malingering or exaggeration because others have manipulated systems to obtain similar accommodations.

The philosopher Michael Walzer's concept of spheres of justice provides a framework for understanding these ethical violations. Walzer argues that different goods should be distributed according to principles appropriate to their nature. Medical care should be allocated based on need, not ability to pay. Educational opportunities should be distributed according to merit and potential, not family wealth. Disability accommodations should be allocated based on functional impairment, not strategic diagnosis-seeking. When diagnostic expansion allows accommodations to be obtained through means other than genuine impairment, it violates the integrity of the distribution sphere, corrupting the principle that should govern allocation.

Consider the situation facing community mental health centers serving low-income populations. These centers employ psychiatrists, psychologists, and social workers who provide services to individuals with serious mental illness, often operating under Medicaid reimbursement at rates substantially below private practice fees. Wait times for initial psychiatric appointments frequently exceed three months. Therapist caseloads commonly reach 60 to 80 active patients. When individuals with mild anxiety or subclinical attentional difficulties seek services at these centers, describing themselves as having clinical disorders based on pop psychology self-diagnosis, they consume appointment slots and therapeutic attention that could serve individuals with schizophrenia, bipolar disorder, or major depressive disorder requiring intensive intervention to prevent hospitalization or suicide.

The triage function of diagnosis becomes critical in this context. A person experiencing transient sadness after a breakup does not require the same therapeutic resources as someone with recurrent major depression who has attempted suicide. A person who sometimes feels nervous before public speaking does not need the same intervention as someone whose panic attacks prevent them from leaving their home. Diagnostic categories exist partly to stratify need, ensuring that limited therapeutic resources flow to those whose suffering and impairment are greatest.

When diagnostic boundaries erode, this stratification fails. Clinics cannot distinguish between patients with severe disorders requiring intensive treatment and patients with mild difficulties manageable through self-help or brief supportive counseling. Everyone presents as "having anxiety" or "having ADHD," rendering the diagnostic labels useless for allocation decisions. Some clinics respond by serving all comers, inevitably providing diluted care to everyone. Others attempt to maintain focus on severe illness but face pressure from patients armed with self-diagnoses demanding services.

The scarcity is not merely financial but also human. Psychiatrists specializing in ADHD develop expertise through years of training and practice. They refine their ability to distinguish genuine executive dysfunction from personality traits, to calibrate medication dosing precisely, to recognize comorbidities that complicate treatment. When these specialists spend appointment time with patients who have mild organizational difficulties rather than genuine ADHD, their expertise is wasted. The patient with severe ADHD who cannot maintain employment despite normal intelligence, who faces eviction because they cannot remember to pay bills, who loses relationships because they cannot regulate emotional responses, waits months for an appointment while the specialist counsels a patient who sometimes procrastinates on tedious tasks.

The ethical principle at stake is captured in the utilitarian calculus of maximizing welfare but also in deontological frameworks emphasizing rights. Individuals with genuine disabilities possess rights to accommodation and treatment that society is obligated to provide. These rights derive from the moral status of severe impairment: when someone cannot access basic opportunities due to biological limitations beyond their control, justice requires society to mitigate those limitations to the extent feasible. These rights create corresponding obligations on resource providers to prioritize genuine need.

When diagnostic expansion allows individuals without genuine disabilities to access resources meant for the disabled, it represents a form of rights violation. The severely impaired student waiting six months for a psychoeducational evaluation while school psychologists assess students with mild difficulties experiences a violation of their right to timely disability determination. The patient with treatment-resistant depression who cannot access a psychiatric appointment for three months while the clinic serves patients with transient situational distress experiences neglect of their right to necessary medical care.

Frances Kamm's philosophical work on scarce resource allocation illuminates the relevant principles. Kamm argues that when resources are scarce, allocation should prioritize those who will benefit most and those whose need is greatest. In medical contexts, this typically means prioritizing life-threatening conditions and severe impairments. A person dying without dialysis has stronger claim to a dialysis machine than someone who could survive without it. Similarly, a student whose disability prevents them from accessing education without accommodation has stronger claim to special education resources than a student who could succeed without support, albeit with more effort.

The challenge is that medical and educational systems struggle to implement such prioritization when diagnostic boundaries blur. If 30% of students claim ADHD diagnoses, how should schools determine which students receive intensive services and which receive minimal support? Without clear functional impairment criteria distinguishing genuine disability from normal-range variation, allocation decisions become arbitrary or default to serving everyone inadequately.

The restoration of ethical resource allocation requires reasserting the connection between diagnosis and functional impairment. Diagnostic labels should be reserved for individuals whose difficulties reach thresholds justifying intervention, whose capacities fall sufficiently below population norms that they cannot access opportunities without support. For educational accommodations, this means requiring documented evidence that disabilities substantially limit learning compared to peers. For pharmacological treatment, this means confirming that symptoms cause significant functional impairment in multiple domains, not merely subjective distress or desire for enhancement.

The implementation of such standards faces resistance because it requires denying diagnoses and accommodations to people who desire them. A student who feels they would benefit from extended test time may experience genuine distress when told they do not qualify. However, the ethical mandate is clear: limited resources must flow to those with greatest need. The mild discomfort of a high-functioning student denied accommodations they do not strictly require cannot outweigh the severe harm to a genuinely disabled student denied necessary support because systems are overwhelmed with questionable cases.

Norman Daniels's work on just health care emphasizes that medical resources should be allocated to maintain normal species functioning, providing individuals with opportunities roughly equal to those available to others. This framework supports restricting accommodations and treatments to individuals whose impairments substantially limit normal functioning. Someone whose attention occasionally wanders maintains normal functioning; they do not require medical intervention. Someone whose attention deficits prevent them from completing education or maintaining employment falls below normal functioning; they merit intervention to restore opportunity.

Society has obligations to provide reasonable accommodations and necessary treatments to individuals with disabilities. These obligations are not infinite; they are bounded by resource constraints and by the principle that accommodations should level the playing field rather than confer advantage. When diagnostic expansion allows accommodations to extend beyond genuinely disabled individuals, the system fails both ethically and practically, consuming finite resources on unnecessary accommodations while leaving truly disabled individuals underserved.

# Part 3: Addressing Rebuttals

# 3.1. The Therapeutic Rebuttal

The phenomenology of suffering contains an element that transcends physical pain or functional limitation. Viktor Frankl, psychiatrist who survived Auschwitz and Dachau, observed that humans possess a fundamental need for their suffering to be recognized and validated by others. In Man's Search for Meaning, Frankl describes how prisoners who felt their anguish went unacknowledged by the world experienced a secondary layer of torment beyond their physical deprivation. This observation, confirmed by decades of subsequent research in clinical psychology, establishes that validation serves genuine psychological needs. When someone struggles with attention, organization, or social interaction, having those struggles recognized as legitimate rather than dismissed as character flaws or laziness provides relief. The contemporary defense of expanded self-diagnosis rests substantially on this foundation: proponents argue that applying diagnostic labels to subclinical experiences offers validation and community to people whose difficulties have been minimized or ignored. This argument merits serious consideration rather than dismissal, for it identifies a real psychological benefit that diagnostic expansion provides. However, the provision of emotional validation cannot supersede the epistemic requirements that give diagnostic categories their meaning and utility.

The validation argument takes several forms in digital discourse. First, individuals describe experiencing relief upon encountering descriptions of ADHD or autism that resonate with their experiences. A person who has always felt scattered, forgetful, or disorganized discovers content explaining these traits as symptoms of ADHD and feels suddenly understood. The realization that others share similar experiences, that these patterns have names and explanations, provides comfort. Second, diagnostic labels facilitate access to communities of others sharing similar experiences. Online forums, support groups, and social media communities organized around diagnostic categories offer belonging and mutual understanding. Third, diagnostic framing recontextualizes struggles as medical conditions rather than personal failings, reducing self-blame and shame.

These benefits possess empirical support. Research by Kendra McLaughlin examining individuals receiving ADHD diagnoses in adulthood documents consistent reports of relief and validation. Participants describe years of feeling inadequate or morally deficient, believing their difficulties reflected laziness or lack of discipline. The diagnosis provided an alternative explanation: their struggles resulted from neurobiological differences rather than character flaws. This reframing reduced self-criticism and hopelessness. Similarly, studies of adults diagnosed with autism spectrum disorder in adulthood, conducted by Sarah Bargiela, reveal that diagnosis often produces profound relief, helping individuals make sense of lifelong experiences of social confusion and sensory overwhelm.

The provision of community represents an equally substantial benefit. Chronic illness research consistently demonstrates that peer support improves coping and reduces distress. Arthur Kleinman's work in medical anthropology emphasizes that illness unfolds not merely as biological pathology but as lived experience shaped by cultural meaning and social response. When patients find others who share their condition, they gain access to experiential knowledge, practical coping strategies, and emotional solidarity that professional treatment alone cannot provide. Cancer patients in support groups show improved psychological adjustment compared to those without peer support. Diabetes patients participating in peer education programs demonstrate better glycemic control.

The diagnostic label serves as the entry ticket to these communities. Online forums typically organize around specific diagnoses, creating spaces for "people with ADHD" or "autistic adults" to connect. Membership implicitly requires identification with the diagnostic category. Someone hesitant to claim a diagnosis may feel excluded from communities that could offer meaningful support. The validation argument thus incorporates both individual psychological benefit and social connection, creating a compelling case that diagnostic expansion serves important therapeutic functions even when it violates traditional diagnostic boundaries.

This argument must be acknowledged as identifying genuine goods. The person who feels validated by adopting an ADHD identity, who finds community among others describing similar experiences, who stops berating themselves for organizational struggles they now understand as symptomatic rather than characterological experiences real psychological benefit. To dismiss these benefits as irrelevant or unimportant would be cruel and phenomenologically dishonest. The question is not whether validation provides value but whether the provision of validation justifies the corruption of diagnostic categories designed to serve epistemic rather than purely therapeutic functions.

The philosopher Bernard Williams distinguished between thick ethical concepts like "cruel" or "courageous," which combine descriptive and evaluative elements, and thin concepts like "good" or "right," which are purely evaluative. Diagnostic labels function as thick concepts: they simultaneously describe patterns of symptoms and dysfunction while evaluating those patterns as pathological rather than normal. The descriptive element grounds the evaluative element. We judge a condition as pathological because it involves functional impairment, not merely because it causes subjective distress.

When diagnostic labels are deployed primarily for their validating or community-building functions, the evaluative element becomes detached from the descriptive element. The label "ADHD" no longer primarily describes a pattern of severe executive dysfunction causing functional impairment but instead functions as a marker of identity and group membership. This detachment represents a category error similar to using scientific terms for their emotional resonance rather than their denotative meaning. Imagine someone claiming to have "Stage 4 cancer" not because they possess malignant tumors but because the phrase validates their experience of suffering and grants access to cancer support communities. The emotional benefit they derive does not justify the misappropriation of a medical category with specific biological meaning.

The Gricean maxims of conversation, articulated by philosopher Paul Grice, specify cooperative principles governing meaningful communication. The maxim of quality demands that speakers make contributions that are true, refraining from asserting what they believe to be false or lack adequate evidence for. The maxim of relation requires that contributions be relevant to conversational purposes. When someone describes themselves as having ADHD primarily for validation and community access rather than because they meet diagnostic criteria, they violate the quality maxim. They assert a medical claim for which they lack adequate evidence, prioritizing emotional benefit over factual accuracy.

The pragma-dialectical approach to argumentation, developed by Frans van Eemeren and Rob Grootendorst, establishes rules for critical discussion aimed at resolving disagreements through rational means. Rule 1, the freedom rule, allows any party to advance or challenge standpoints. Rule 2, the burden of proof rule, requires parties to defend their standpoints when challenged. Rule 5, the unexpressed premise rule, requires parties to accept responsibility for implicit commitments of their stated positions. Most relevant here is Rule 8, the validity rule, which demands that reasoning be logically valid or capable of being made valid through explicit articulation of missing premises.

When someone claims to have ADHD based on subjective identification rather than diagnostic assessment, they implicitly commit to the premise that ADHD diagnosis is legitimately established through self-identification. This premise cannot withstand critical scrutiny. Medical diagnoses are not performative speech acts that become true through assertion. They are empirical claims about biological or psychological states, requiring evidence from systematic assessment. The validation argument attempts to sidestep this epistemic requirement by shifting terrain from truth claims to therapeutic utility, but this shift violates argumentation rules by refusing to defend the factual basis of diagnostic claims.

The sociologist Erving Goffman analyzed how stigmatized identities are managed in social interaction. In Stigma: Notes on the Management of Spoiled Identity, Goffman describes how individuals with discredited identities navigate tension between concealment and disclosure. Medical diagnoses of psychiatric conditions carry stigma, marking individuals as defective or abnormal. Goffman would predict that many people would avoid psychiatric labels to escape stigmatization. The contemporary phenomenon of voluntary diagnostic adoption appears paradoxical from this framework.

The resolution lies in recognizing that diagnostic labels now provide benefits that outweigh their stigmatic costs in certain social contexts. Within online communities organized around neurodiversity frameworks, ADHD and autism labels confer positive identity rather than stigma. They signal membership in a marginalized group, authenticate personal struggles as medically legitimate, and provide narrative coherence to fragmented life experiences. The therapeutic benefits Goffman could not have foreseen emerge from subcultural revaluations of psychiatric categories, transforming them from marks of deficiency into badges of authentic selfhood.

However, this transformation depends on a tacit bait-and-switch. The diagnostic categories derive their validating power from their status as medical constructs identifying genuine neurobiological differences. If ADHD were understood as an arbitrary label people adopt for community and validation, it would lose its capacity to recontextualize struggles as non-characterological. The validation works because the diagnosis implies "My brain works differently through no fault of my own," not "I have chosen to identify with a community." But if diagnostic categories are to maintain their medical authority and validating power, they must remain grounded in empirical criteria rather than self-identification.

The philosopher J.L. Austin distinguished between constative utterances, which describe states of affairs and can be true or false, and performative utterances, which perform actions through their enunciation and are felicitous or infelicitous rather than true or false. "I promise to meet you tomorrow" is performative; it enacts a promise rather than describing a pre-existing state. "I have ADHD" appears grammatically similar to performative utterances of identity like "I am a patriot" or "I am a Christian", which can be made true through authentic self-identification. However, ideally, medical diagnoses are constative rather than performative. They ought to describe purported biological or psychological facts, making them subject to verification rather than matters of self-determination.

The validation argument attempts to treat diagnostic utterances as performative, as acts of self-identification that cannot be challenged without violating autonomy. This represents a speech act category error. While identity claims like religious or political affiliation are indeed performative and self-authenticating, medical diagnoses remain constative. Someone cannot make themselves diabetic by sincerely identifying as such. The validation benefits of diagnostic self-identification do not transform medical categories into matters of personal choice.

Ian Hacking's concept of "making up people" illuminates how diagnostic categories can become self-fulfilling through social processes. Hacking argues that human kinds differ from natural kinds because humans classified under a category can become aware of that classification and modify their behavior accordingly, which then changes the category itself. His canonical example involves multiple personality disorder, whose diagnostic criteria and symptomatic presentations evolved through interaction between clinicians, patients, and popular culture. Patients learned what multiple personality was supposed to look like and enacted those presentations, while clinicians refined diagnostic criteria based on observed presentations.

ADHD and autism appear to be undergoing similar looping effects. As diagnostic categories enter popular discourse, people learn the symptom profiles and begin interpreting their own experiences through diagnostic frameworks. Someone who previously understood themselves as disorganized learns that ADHD involves disorganization and begins attributing all instances of forgetfulness to ADHD rather than to universal human fallibility. The category shapes experience, and altered experience reinforces identification with the category.

However, Hacking's looping effects describe what happens, not what should happen. The fact that diagnostic categories can be socially constructed through interaction between classifiers and classified does not mean that epistemic standards are irrelevant. Natural kinds in biology and medicine are not immune to social construction, but they remain tethered to objective reality through empirical validation. The concept "autism" has undoubtedly been shaped by social processes, but genuinely autistic individuals exist independently of the category's social construction. A three-year-old who does not speak, does not make eye contact, and engages in repetitive behaviors manifests real developmental differences, however much the precise boundaries and conceptualization of autism as a diagnostic category reflect social factors.

The validation argument prioritizes the therapeutic effects of labeling over the epistemic function of accurate classification. This prioritization reflects a broader cultural trend toward therapeutic understandings of selfhood, identified by sociologist Philip Rieff in The Triumph of the Therapeutic. Rieff argued that Western culture increasingly interprets human experience through psychological rather than moral or religious frameworks, prioritizing emotional well-being over adherence to normative standards. From this therapeutic perspective, if diagnostic labels make people feel better by providing validation and community, the accuracy of those labels becomes secondary.

Yet medicine cannot function on purely therapeutic grounds. The physician who tells a patient they have cancer when they do not, because the patient finds the diagnosis validating or wants to join cancer support communities, commits ethical and professional violations regardless of any psychological benefit the patient derives. Medical truth claims must be constrained by evidence rather than therapeutic utility. Diagnostic categories serve practical functions beyond emotional validation: they guide treatment decisions, predict prognosis, allocate resources, and structure research. When diagnostic labels become detached from empirical criteria and deployed for purely validating purposes, these practical functions fail.

The harm extends to patient advocacy and collective credibility. Disability rights movements achieved legal protections and social accommodations through sustained advocacy demonstrating that disabled individuals face genuine barriers requiring societal response. The Americans with Disabilities Act passed in 1990 partly because advocates effectively communicated that disabilities involve functional limitations beyond individual control, justifying reasonable accommodations. This advocacy succeeded because it was grounded in demonstrable impairment affecting specific individuals in identifiable ways.

When diagnostic categories expand to include subclinical presentations primarily for validation and community purposes, advocacy becomes epistemically compromised. If large numbers of people claiming ADHD diagnoses do not experience functional impairment, skeptics can dismiss accommodation requests as preference-seeking rather than disability remediation. The student who genuinely needs extended time because severe reading disability prevents them from accessing test material within standard time becomes indistinguishable from the student who would simply prefer extra time to check answers more carefully. Collective advocacy loses credibility when the boundaries of the advocated-for group become unclear.

Naomi Scheman's philosophical work on empathy and testimony emphasizes that marginalized groups depend on having their testimony believed by dominant groups to achieve recognition and accommodation. When women report experiences of sexual harassment, when people of color describe experiences of discrimination, credibility becomes crucial. If listeners doubt the veracity of testimony, the described experiences cannot prompt social response. Disability advocacy similarly depends on credibility: society must believe that described impairments are real and severe enough to warrant accommodation.

The inflation of diagnostic categories through self-identification without functional impairment undermines this credibility. When significant numbers of people adopt diagnostic labels primarily for validation and community rather than to describe genuine disability, it creates suspicion that all such claims are similarly grounded in desire for validation rather than objective impairment. The person with severe executive dysfunction whose ADHD prevents them from maintaining employment suffers when others doubt their diagnosis because diagnostic labels have been diluted through expansive application.

The tragedy is that the validation seekers and the genuinely impaired face different problems requiring different solutions. People experiencing mild organizational difficulties or social awkwardness who seek validation need recognition that their struggles are real without pathologizing normal human variation. Appropriate responses include normalizing discussions of personality differences, reducing stigma around asking for help with executive function skills, and creating communities around shared temperamental traits rather than diagnostic categories. Someone low in conscientiousness can find community with others who share that personality profile without claiming ADHD. Someone high in introversion and sensory sensitivity can find community with others sharing those traits without claiming autism.

By contrast, people with genuine functional impairments need accurate diagnosis leading to effective treatment and appropriate accommodation. Their validation comes not from labels per se but from having their real limitations recognized and addressed. A child whose ADHD is so severe they cannot learn in a regular classroom needs intensive intervention, not merely validation. A diagnosis that accurately identifies their impairment provides validation precisely because it is accurate, because it reflects reality rather than serving as a comforting narrative.

The philosopher Miranda Fricker's concept of epistemic injustice distinguishes testimonial injustice, where speakers are not believed due to prejudice, from hermeneutical injustice, where speakers lack conceptual resources to articulate their experiences. People experiencing subclinical difficulties may face hermeneutical injustice: our culture lacks adequate non-pathological language for describing variation in attention, sensory sensitivity, or social communication. The response to hermeneutical injustice is developing richer ordinary vocabulary, not misappropriating clinical categories.

We need language that validates difficulties without medicalizing them. Concepts like "highly sensitive person," "introverted," "low in conscientiousness," "detail-oriented," "need for routine" provide such language. These terms describe real individual differences, acknowledge that some patterns can create challenges, and facilitate community among people sharing similar profiles, all without invoking pathology or claiming disability status. The therapeutic functions currently served by expansive diagnostic self-identification could be served by such vocabulary if it received cultural validation.

Speakers have obligations to make accurate claims in domains where truth matters practically. This obligation applies particularly strongly to medical claims, where inaccuracy can lead to inappropriate treatment, resource misallocation, and erosion of diagnostic systems. The obligation does not require perfect certainty but does require reasonable evidence and good-faith engagement with epistemic standards. Someone who claims to have ADHD without seeking professional assessment or meeting diagnostic criteria violates this obligation regardless of the psychological benefits they derive from the claim.

The restoration of diagnostic integrity requires decoupling validation from diagnosis. Validation should flow from recognition of genuine struggles and provision of appropriate support, not from assignment of pathological labels. Someone experiencing mild executive function difficulties deserves validation, support, and access to organizational strategies. They do not deserve or require a diagnosis of ADHD unless their difficulties reach impairment thresholds. Similarly, someone with intense sensory sensitivities deserves validation and accommodation of their sensory needs. They do not require an autism diagnosis unless their difficulties create pervasive functional limitations across social communication and behavior domains.

The therapeutic functions of community and validation can be preserved while restoring epistemic rigor to diagnostic practice. This requires cultural work: developing and promoting non-pathological language for human variation, creating communities organized around traits rather than diagnoses, and emphasizing that validation does not require medical framing. It also requires clinical work: ensuring that genuinely impaired individuals receive timely diagnosis and that diagnostic processes distinguish impairment from normal variation. Most fundamentally, it requires philosophical clarity about the proper function of diagnostic categories and the limits of therapeutic justifications for epistemic compromise.

## 3.2. The Anti-Stigma Rebuttal

The anti-stigma movement in mental health traces its modern formulation to the work of sociologist Erving Goffman, whose 1963 book Stigma analyzed how societies mark certain attributes as discrediting, transforming individuals possessing those attributes into devalued social categories. Goffman documented how psychiatric diagnoses function as master statuses, overriding other aspects of identity and subjecting individuals to discrimination in employment, housing, and social relationships. The subsequent decades witnessed sustained efforts to reduce mental health stigma through public education campaigns, legislative protections, and cultural advocacy. The National Alliance on Mental Illness, founded in 1979, has worked to reframe mental illness as brain disease rather than character weakness, arguing that biological conceptualizations reduce blame and prejudice. More recently, the neurodiversity movement, articulated by sociologist Judy Singer in 1998 and popularized by journalist Steve Silberman's 2015 book NeuroTribes, has reframed conditions like autism and ADHD as natural variations rather than deficits, celebrating cognitive differences rather than pathologizing them.

Contemporary advocates for diagnostic expansion argue that broadening the boundaries of categories like ADHD and autism reduces stigma by normalizing these conditions. The reasoning follows an intuitive logic: if 40% of the population qualifies as neurodivergent rather than 5%, the conditions become common rather than aberrant, familiar rather than frightening. When everyone knows multiple people with ADHD, when the category includes successful professionals and creative individuals alongside those with severe impairments, the diagnosis loses its association with incompetence or abnormality. The stigma attached to being diagnosed dissipates as the diagnosis becomes ubiquitous. This argument has achieved wide acceptance in online advocacy communities, where expansive definitions of neurodivergence are defended explicitly as stigma-reduction strategies.

The empirical question is whether diagnostic expansion actually reduces stigma or whether it produces unintended consequences that worsen outcomes for the most severely impaired. The limited research addressing this question suggests that the relationship between prevalence and stigma is more complex than the normalization hypothesis predicts. Contact theory, developed by psychologist Gordon Allport in his 1954 book The Nature of Prejudice, proposes that interpersonal contact with stigmatized groups reduces prejudice under certain conditions: equal status between groups, common goals, intergroup cooperation, and institutional support.

Applied to mental health stigma, contact theory predicts that familiarity with people who have psychiatric diagnoses should reduce negative attitudes.

Studies testing contact theory in mental health contexts yield mixed results. Patrick Corrigan's research demonstrates that contact with people who have serious mental illness can reduce stigma, but the effect depends on the nature of the contact. Superficial contact or contact with individuals whose symptoms are severe and disruptive can actually increase stigma by confirming negative stereotypes. Effective stigma reduction requires sustained contact with individuals whose psychiatric conditions are well-managed, who demonstrate competence in social and occupational domains, and who disconfirm stereotypes about dangerousness or incompetence.

The relevance to diagnostic expansion becomes clear when we consider what happens as diagnostic categories broaden to include highly functional individuals. If ADHD expands to encompass successful entrepreneurs who credit their "ADHD" with creative thinking and risk-taking, while also including individuals whose executive dysfunction prevents them from maintaining employment, the public encounters two radically different presentations under the same label. Contact with the successful entrepreneur might indeed reduce stigma, as the public sees that "ADHD" is compatible with achievement. However, this contact may simultaneously trivialize the condition, leading to the conclusion that ADHD is not a serious impairment but merely a personality variant or even an advantage in certain contexts.

The trivialization paradox emerges from this dynamic: as diagnostic categories expand to include mild presentations and highly functional individuals, the perceived severity and legitimacy of the condition decreases. The public concludes that if most people with ADHD function normally or even excel, then ADHD cannot be a genuine disability requiring accommodation or treatment. The person with severe executive dysfunction whose ADHD prevents them from completing basic tasks then faces increased skepticism. Others assume their struggles reflect lack of effort rather than genuine impairment because the category now encompasses so many people who manage perfectly well.

This paradox finds empirical support in research on disability accommodation skepticism. A 2019 study by Nicole Ditchman examining employer attitudes toward psychiatric disabilities found that employers expressed more skepticism about the legitimacy of ADHD accommodations than about accommodations for physical disabilities or sensory impairments. Qualitative interviews revealed that employers frequently knew multiple people claiming ADHD diagnoses who performed well without accommodations, leading them to view accommodation requests as preference-seeking rather than disability remediation. The expansion of the diagnostic category had undermined rather than enhanced perceived legitimacy.

The mechanism underlying this effect relates to category-based inference. When people encounter a category label like "ADHD," they form prototype representations based on their exposure to category exemplars. If most exemplars they encounter are mildly affected and highly functional, the prototype becomes "ADHD is not particularly impairing." This prototype then influences how they interpret and respond to all individuals bearing the label, including those whose impairments are severe. The severely impaired individual is judged against a prototype that does not match their experience, leading observers to conclude they are exaggerating, malingering, or simply not trying hard enough.

Social psychologist Susan Fiske's work on stereotypes and prejudice demonstrates that category perception operates through a process of abstraction, where exposure to category members generates schematic representations that guide subsequent judgments. When a category is heterogeneous, containing members with vastly different characteristics, perceivers tend to focus on the most common or salient exemplars in forming their schema. If diagnostic expansion ensures that the most common exemplars of ADHD are mildly affected individuals maintaining normal functioning, the schema for ADHD will not include severe impairment, making genuinely disabled individuals seem atypical or questionable.

The neurodiversity movement's reframing of autism and ADHD as differences rather than disorders accelerates this trivialization. The concept of neurodiversity, while valuable in some respects, carries an implicit message that neurological variations are neutral differences in information processing rather than impairments requiring remediation. Temple Grandin, autistic animal scientist and prominent neurodiversity advocate, exemplifies this framing: her autism confers advantages in visual thinking that contribute to her professional success. Grandin has repeatedly emphasized that autism involves different rather than deficient cognition.

However, Grandin's autism is relatively mild in some respects. She acquired spoken language, completed advanced education, and maintains independent living and employment. Her public visibility makes her a salient exemplar of autism, shaping how the public conceptualizes the condition. Meanwhile, the approximately 30% of autistic individuals who remain minimally verbal into adulthood, the majority who never achieve competitive employment, and the substantial fraction who require lifelong supported living become invisible in public discourse. The category "autism" comes to evoke Temple Grandin rather than the profoundly impaired individuals who constitute a significant portion of the diagnostic category.

The parents of severely impaired autistic children have voiced increasing concern about this dynamic. Amy Lutz, mother of a son with severe autism who engages in self-injurious behavior and requires constant supervision, has written extensively about how neurodiversity framing marginalizes families dealing with profound disability. She argues that the celebration of mild autism as mere difference trivializes the struggles of families managing aggression, self-injury, and complete dependence. When autism advocacy focuses on celebrating neurodiversity and opposing the search for causes or cures, families of severely affected children feel abandoned by a movement that no longer acknowledges their reality.

The trivialization paradox operates through multiple mechanisms beyond prototype formation. One mechanism involves comparative judgment. When people assess the severity of an impairment, they implicitly compare it to reference points drawn from their experience. If someone's reference point for ADHD is an organized, high-achieving friend who claims the diagnosis, they will judge genuine executive dysfunction against that reference point and find it insufficiently severe to warrant special consideration. The expansion of diagnostic categories shifts reference points in ways that disadvantage the severely impaired.

Another mechanism involves resource allocation decisions by institutions and policymakers. When a condition is perceived as common and mild, it receives lower priority for research funding, treatment development, and accommodation provision. Hannah Decker's history of DSM development documents how diagnostic prevalence affects research priorities. Rare conditions attract limited research interest because they affect few people. Common conditions attract interest proportional to their perceived public health burden. However, if a condition is simultaneously common and perceived as mild, it falls into a dead zone: affecting too many people for individualized intensive intervention but seeming insufficiently serious to justify major public health investment.

ADHD appears to be entering this zone. As prevalence estimates have risen from 3% to 10% or higher in some studies, and as public discourse increasingly frames ADHD as a common variation rather than serious disorder, research funding has not kept pace with prevalence. The National Institute of Mental Health's research budget for ADHD was approximately $100 million in 2022, less than funding for schizophrenia despite ADHD's dramatically higher prevalence. The relative underfunding likely reflects perceptions that ADHD is not a serious condition, perceptions fostered partly by diagnostic expansion and normalization rhetoric.

The philosopher Nancy Fraser's work on recognition and redistribution illuminates the tension between stigma reduction and resource allocation. Fraser argues that social justice requires both cultural recognition, dismantling stigma and devaluation of marginalized groups, and material redistribution, ensuring that disadvantaged groups receive adequate resources. These two goals can conflict: strategies that promote recognition may undermine redistribution, and vice versa. Applied to disability, efforts to reduce stigma by normalizing conditions and celebrating difference may inadvertently reduce the perceived need for resource allocation to support those who cannot function without intensive intervention.

The deaf community provides an instructive parallel. Deaf culture advocates have successfully reframed deafness as linguistic and cultural difference rather than pathological deficit. This recognition-based strategy has reduced stigma and promoted deaf pride. However, it has also complicated efforts to secure resources for cochlear implants and spoken language therapy, interventions that some deaf children need to access mainstream educational and employment opportunities. The celebration of deaf culture as complete unto itself can be interpreted as implying that deaf individuals require no special resources, harming those whose life circumstances make sign language insufficient for their needs.

The ADHD and autism communities face similar tensions. Celebrating neurodivergence as valuable difference reduces stigma for high-functioning individuals who experience their conditions as personality variants. However, it obscures the reality that severe ADHD and autism involve profound impairments requiring intensive, costly interventions. The child with severe autism who engages in dangerous self-injury, the adult with ADHD who cannot maintain employment despite normal intelligence, these individuals need the public to understand their conditions as serious disabilities warranting substantial support. Trivialization through normalization actively harms them.

The concept of "spoiled identity" from Goffman's stigma theory takes on new meaning in this context. Goffman described how stigmatized attributes spoil identity by becoming master statuses that override other characteristics. The traditional anti-stigma strategy aimed to unspoil identity by demonstrating that people with psychiatric conditions possess other valued attributes. However, diagnostic expansion creates a different problem: the identity becomes so diluted that it ceases to communicate meaningful information. An ADHD diagnosis no longer signals specific impairments requiring specific accommodations; it signals membership in a vaguely defined group encompassing everything from severe disability to mild personality quirks.

This dilution spoils identity in a different way: it renders the diagnosis simultaneously over-determining and under-informative. The person who discloses an ADHD diagnosis faces stereotypes drawn from the public's heterogeneous experience with the category, stereotypes that may bear no relationship to their actual impairments. Simultaneously, the diagnosis fails to convey necessary information about what accommodations they require, leading to the need for extensive additional explanation that undermines the communicative efficiency diagnoses should provide.

Philosopher Alasdair MacIntyre's concept of practices and internal goods offers a framework for understanding what goes wrong. MacIntyre argues that social practices like medicine possess internal goods, standards of excellence intrinsic to the practice that define success. For diagnostic practice, internal goods include accuracy, specificity, and predictive validity. These goods serve the practice's purpose: identifying who requires intervention and predicting response to treatment. External goods like prestige or income are important but should remain subordinate to internal goods.

When diagnostic categories are expanded primarily to achieve external goods like stigma reduction or community building, internal goods are sacrificed. A diagnostic system optimized for stigma reduction looks very different from one optimized for accuracy and predictive validity. The former applies diagnoses broadly to normalize conditions; the latter restricts diagnoses to individuals meeting clear impairment criteria. Contemporary advocacy increasingly prioritizes external goods over internal goods, corrupting the practice of diagnosis.

The harm becomes clearest in situations where accurate diagnosis matters most. Consider a young adult seeking disability benefits due to inability to maintain employment. The Social Security Administration's disability determination process requires evidence that the applicant's condition prevents them from engaging in substantial gainful activity. When ADHD has been reframed as common neurodiversity compatible with normal functioning, adjudicators view ADHD claims skeptically. The applicant whose executive dysfunction genuinely prevents them from maintaining employment faces the burden of proving that their ADHD is "real" in a context where the diagnosis has been thoroughly trivialized.

Data from Social Security disability determination support this concern. Approval rates for claims based on ADHD are substantially lower than for most other conditions, typically below 20% at initial determination. Adjudicators frequently deny claims on grounds that ADHD is not severe enough to prevent all work, citing examples of successful individuals with ADHD. The claimant who cannot function faces the consequences of a diagnostic category that has been expanded to include high-functioning individuals.

The trivialization paradox also manifests in educational contexts. The Individuals with Disabilities Education Act requires that schools provide Free Appropriate Public Education to students with disabilities, including those with ADHD that substantially limits learning. However, as ADHD diagnoses have proliferated and the condition has been normalized, schools have become increasingly resistant to providing intensive services. A 2018 Government Accountability Office report documented that many school districts interpret "appropriate" narrowly, providing minimal accommodations while reserving intensive services for students with more obviously severe disabilities.

School personnel interviewed for the report expressed skepticism about ADHD's severity, noting that many students with ADHD diagnoses perform adequately without services. This skepticism likely reflects exposure to the many students diagnosed under expansive criteria who function well academically. The student with severe ADHD whose reading comprehension and math problem-solving fail despite adequate intelligence because they cannot sustain attention long enough to complete multi-step tasks suffers from this skepticism, receiving inadequate services because their diagnosis has been devalued through over-application.

The solution to stigma cannot lie in trivializing genuine disability. The philosopher Elizabeth Anderson's work on democratic equality proposes an alternative framework. Anderson argues that equality requires not eliminating differences but ensuring that differences do not generate oppressive social hierarchies. Applied to disability, this suggests that stigma reduction should aim not to minimize or normalize disability but to ensure that disabled individuals have equal access to opportunities and are treated with equal respect despite genuine impairments.

This approach maintains diagnostic rigor while combating stigma. ADHD diagnosis remains restricted to individuals with significant functional impairment, preserving the category's seriousness and specificity. Anti-stigma efforts focus on changing attitudes toward disability itself, promoting understanding that impairment is compatible with dignity and worth. The public learns that people with ADHD face genuine challenges requiring accommodation, not that ADHD is just another personality type requiring no special consideration.

The neuroscientist Robert Sapolsky's public communication about biological bases of behavior illustrates this approach. Sapolsky emphasizes that neurobiological explanations for behavior do not trivialize the behavior or eliminate the need for response. A violent individual whose aggression stems from amygdala hyperreactivity still requires intervention, not celebration of their neurological difference. Similarly, an individual whose executive dysfunction stems from prefrontal-striatal circuit inefficiency still requires treatment and accommodation, not merely reframing of their condition as neurodiversity.

Advocates have obligations to represent their constituencies accurately. Disability advocacy that obscures the severity of impairment experienced by the most affected individuals betrays those individuals in service of broader normalization goals. The severely autistic child who requires constant supervision is not served by advocacy that celebrates autism as mere cognitive difference. The adult with ADHD who cannot maintain employment is not served by advocacy that frames ADHD as entrepreneurial thinking style.

Effective stigma reduction requires acknowledging the reality of severe impairment while insisting that impairment does not diminish human worth. This acknowledgment is compatible with celebrating the achievements of high-functioning individuals with disabilities, but it cannot allow those achievements to obscure the struggles of the severely impaired. The category boundaries must remain calibrated to genuine disability, even if this means that mildly affected individuals do not receive the validation of diagnostic labels. Their validation must come from other sources: recognition of their struggles as real without pathologizing them, access to support and accommodations through non-medical channels, and cultural acknowledgment that human variation in attention and social cognition does not require diagnostic framing to warrant respect and consideration.

# Part 4: Synthesis

# 4.1. A Call for Conceptual Honesty

The physician Atul Gawande, in his 2002 book Complications: A Surgeon's Notes on an Imperfect Science, describes the terror of diagnostic uncertainty in acute medical situations. A patient arrives at the emergency department with abdominal pain. The differential diagnosis spans from benign gastroenteritis requiring only supportive care to perforated viscus requiring immediate surgery. The stakes are existential: misdiagnosis in either direction can be fatal. Too quick to diagnose appendicitis and operate, and the surgeon inflicts unnecessary harm on a patient with viral illness. Too slow to recognize surgical abdomen, and the patient dies of septic shock. Medicine's entire apparatus of diagnostic precision exists because these distinctions matter desperately. The language we use to categorize human suffering is not merely descriptive but interventional, determining who receives which treatments and predicting who faces which futures. When diagnostic language loses precision, it loses its capacity to guide action, becoming noise rather than signal.

The preceding analysis has established multiple converging lines of argument demonstrating that contemporary pop psychology has initiated a process of diagnostic degradation that threatens the conceptual infrastructure of mental health care. The continuum fallacy transforms dimensional traits into categorical diseases, ignoring the statistical reality that clinical diagnoses identify the extreme tails of normal distributions where functional impairment becomes severe. The loss of predictive validity shows that diluted diagnostic categories no longer forecast the outcomes that justify clinical attention: educational failure, occupational disability, relationship dissolution, suicide risk. The violation of conceptual parsimony introduces unnecessary pathological entities where ordinary psychological vocabulary would suffice. The misallocation of scarce resources diverts specialized services from the severely impaired to the subclinically affected, violating principles of distributive justice. The therapeutic and anti-stigma rationales for diagnostic expansion, while identifying real psychological needs, cannot supersede epistemic requirements without corrupting the scientific and clinical utility of diagnostic categories.

These arguments converge on a single conclusion: the expansion of clinical diagnostic labels to encompass subclinical presentations represents not democratic access to medical validation but conceptual pseudomedicine, a practice that appropriates the language and authority of medical science while abandoning the empirical standards that give that language meaning. This conclusion carries profound implications for how we understand and respond to human psychological variation, implications that extend beyond academic debates into the lived experiences of genuinely impaired individuals whose access to care and accommodation depends on maintaining diagnostic clarity.

The term pseudomedicine traditionally denotes practices that mimic medical authority without scientific foundation: homeopathy's invocation of biological mechanisms to explain treatments with no active ingredients, chiropractic's theories of subluxation unsupported by anatomical evidence, energy healing's appropriation of physics terminology to describe undetectable forces. These practices share a common structure: they deploy scientific language to gain credibility while violating the empirical standards that scientific language presupposes. The harm they cause operates through multiple mechanisms. Direct harm occurs when patients forego effective treatments for pseudoscientific alternatives. Indirect harm occurs through resource consumption, as healthcare systems expend money on ineffective treatments. Cultural harm occurs through erosion of scientific literacy and public trust in evidence-based medicine.

Conceptual pseudomedicine operates through analogous mechanisms but targets the linguistic and categorical infrastructure of medicine rather than specific treatments. When diagnostic terms are applied without adherence to validated criteria, when functional impairment requirements are ignored, when self-diagnosis substitutes for systematic assessment, the resulting practice mimics medical diagnosis while abandoning its empirical foundations. The language of pathology is invoked, but the standards that give pathological categories their meaning are discarded. This represents pseudomedicine at the conceptual level, degrading diagnostic categories themselves rather than promoting specific fraudulent treatments.

The harm this conceptual degradation causes is multifaceted and substantial. At the individual level, people who adopt diagnostic labels without meeting clinical criteria may pursue unnecessary treatments carrying genuine risks. Stimulant medications prescribed for questionable ADHD diagnoses expose patients to cardiovascular side effects, abuse potential, and psychological dependence. Methylphenidate raises blood pressure and heart rate through its sympathomimetic effects on alpha and beta adrenergic receptors. While these risks are justified when treating genuine ADHD that would otherwise cause severe functional impairment, the risk-benefit calculus shifts dramatically when treating subclinical attentional variation that could be managed through behavioral strategies.

Casey Schwartz's 2018 book In the Mind Fields documents the amphetamine use trajectory among her peer group at elite universities. Students obtain ADHD diagnoses strategically, beginning stimulant use for academic performance enhancement. Many develop tolerance, requiring escalating doses to maintain effects. Some transition to non-prescribed stimulants when medical providers become uncomfortable with dose escalation. Schwartz describes the psychological transformation that occurs: tasks previously manageable through discipline become impossible without pharmaceutical augmentation. The medication that was supposed to correct a deficit creates dependency that impairs natural executive function. While Schwartz's account is anecdotal, controlled studies demonstrate that chronic stimulant exposure in individuals without ADHD can produce lasting alterations in dopamine receptor density and reward circuitry function.

At the systemic level, the flooding of diagnostic categories with subclinical presentations overwhelms support systems designed for the genuinely disabled. The analysis in Chapter 4 documented how special education resources, psychiatric services, and disability accommodations become scarce goods when demand exceeds supply through diagnostic inflation. The child with profound autism who needs intensive behavioral intervention waits months because therapists are serving children with mild social awkwardness. The adult with treatment-resistant major depression cannot access a psychiatrist because clinics are filled with patients experiencing transient situational distress who learned to describe their sadness as clinical depression. The college student whose reading disability requires assistive technology cannot obtain timely evaluation because school disability offices are processing hundreds of accommodation requests from students seeking competitive advantage.

This resource diversion represents not merely inefficiency but injustice. The philosopher John Rawls articulated the difference principle: social and economic inequalities are justifiable only when they benefit the least advantaged members of society. Applied to healthcare resource allocation, this principle demands that limited resources flow preferentially to those most impaired, those whose capacity for normal functioning is most compromised. When diagnostic expansion allows mildly affected individuals to access resources meant for the severely disabled, the least advantaged are harmed to benefit the moderately or minimally affected. This violates basic principles of medical ethics and distributive justice.

The cultural harm operates through mechanisms analyzed in Chapter 6: trivialization of genuine disability through normalization of diagnostic labels.

When a diagnostic category encompasses both individuals whose impairments prevent them from maintaining employment or completing education and individuals who function normally but find the label validating, the category loses its capacity to communicate severity and need. Employers become skeptical of accommodation requests when "ADHD" might mean anything from severe executive dysfunction to mild distractibility. Educators resist providing intensive services when "autism" might describe a socially successful adult who prefers routine or a minimally verbal child who requires constant supervision. The severely impaired individual's genuine needs become invisible, submerged in a heterogeneous category dominated numerically by the mildly affected or unaffected.

This trivialization extends to research domains. The psychiatrist Thomas Insel, reflecting on his tenure leading the National Institute of Mental Health, has expressed frustration that psychiatric research makes slow progress partly because diagnostic heterogeneity obscures genuine biological signals. Studies enrolling participants based on DSM criteria gather samples containing individuals with fundamentally different underlying pathologies, different etiologies, different treatment responses. The resulting data become uninterpretable noise. Genetic studies searching for ADHD risk variants find effect sizes so small as to be clinically meaningless partly because samples include substantial numbers of people without genuine ADHD whose genetic architecture differs from truly affected individuals. Neuroimaging studies comparing ADHD patients to controls show inconsistent results partly because the "ADHD" group contains heterogeneous presentations including subclinical cases. The cumulative effect is that research progress stalls, treatment development slows, and genuinely impaired individuals wait longer for effective interventions.

The philosopher of science Thomas Kuhn distinguished normal science, which operates within established paradigms using accepted methods and concepts, from revolutionary science, which challenges and reconstructs paradigms when accumulated anomalies render them untenable. Psychiatric nosology is not undergoing Kuhnian revolution but something more insidious: conceptual decay through progressive relaxation of standards. The paradigm itself remains nominally intact, diagnostic manuals still specify criteria, but enforcement of those criteria erodes through social pressure, cultural trends, and economic incentives. The result is not dramatic paradigm shift but gradual loss of diagnostic meaning, a process more akin to language degradation than scientific revolution.

George Orwell's 1946 essay "Politics and the English Language" analyzed how political corruption produces linguistic corruption, as clear language becomes dangerous to those with interests in obscuring truth. Orwell argued that unclear language facilitates unclear thinking, which in turn enables unjust practices. The degradation of diagnostic language follows an analogous pattern. When diagnostic terms lose clear referents, when they can be applied to nearly anyone based on subjective identification, they cease to serve truth-tracking functions. This linguistic corruption serves certain interests: pharmaceutical companies benefit from expanded patient populations, online content creators benefit from viral content about relatable symptoms, individuals seeking validation or accommodations benefit from accessible diagnoses. However, it profoundly harms those who need diagnostic categories to function as precise tools identifying genuine pathology.

The path forward requires rejecting the false choice between diagnostic rigor and compassionate recognition of human suffering. We need not choose between maintaining strict diagnostic boundaries and validating people's struggles. Both imperatives can be honored through conceptual discipline and linguistic precision. Clinical diagnoses should be reserved for presentations meeting clear functional impairment criteria, maintaining their role as scientific and medical tools. Simultaneously, culture must develop richer non-pathological vocabulary for discussing human psychological variation, acknowledging that traits like distractibility, sensory sensitivity, social awkwardness, and organizational difficulty exist on continua and can create challenges without reaching pathological thresholds.

The psychologist Jerome Kagan's work on temperament provides a model for such vocabulary.[1] Kagan identified behavioral inhibition as a stable temperamental trait present from infancy, characterized by heightened reactivity to novelty and unfamiliarity. Approximately 15-20% of children exhibit high behavioral inhibition, showing distress in novel situations, wariness of strangers, and cautious engagement with new environments. This trait predicts increased risk for anxiety disorders but is not itself pathological. Most behaviorally inhibited children develop normally, learning to manage their temperamental tendencies without treatment. Kagan's framework acknowledges real individual differences, validates that these differences can create challenges, and provides non-pathological language for discussing them.

We need similar frameworks for traits currently being pathologized through diagnostic expansion. Normal variations in attentional control,

---

[1] Cynthia Garcia Coll et al., "Behavioral Inhibition in Young Children," *Child Development* 55, no. 3 (1984): 1005–19, https://doi.org/10.2307/1130152.

organizational capacity, sensory processing, and social communication exist across populations and can be discussed using psychological vocabulary that does not invoke disease. Someone low in trait self-control, as measured by personality psychologists like Roy Baumeister, will struggle with impulse regulation and delayed gratification without necessarily having ADHD. Someone high in openness to experience, one of the Big Five personality dimensions, may find routine boring and seek novelty without meeting criteria for attention deficit disorder. Someone with heightened sensory processing sensitivity, as studied by Elaine Aron, may find intense stimulation overwhelming without having sensory processing disorder.

This linguistic reframing serves multiple functions. It validates struggles as real without pathologizing them. It provides community and identity around shared traits without requiring diagnostic labels. It preserves clinical diagnoses for individuals whose difficulties reach impairment thresholds. It maintains the scientific integrity of psychiatric nosology while expanding cultural capacity to discuss human variation with nuance and compassion.

The implementation of this reframing requires coordinated effort across multiple domains. Medical education must emphasize the distinction between symptoms and syndromes, teaching future clinicians to distinguish common human experiences from clinical disorders. Diagnostic training should stress functional impairment as the decisive criterion separating pathology from normal variation. Clinicians should be prepared to tell patients that their struggles are real and deserving of support without meeting thresholds for formal diagnosis, providing validation without diagnostic labels.

Public health communication must shift from normalizing mental illness through prevalence inflation to accurately representing both the reality of severe mental illness and the frequency of milder psychological difficulties. Anti-stigma campaigns should emphasize that mental illness involves genuine impairment requiring treatment, not that everyone has mental illness. Educational materials should distinguish clinical depression from sadness, clinical anxiety from nervousness, ADHD from distractibility. The goal should be accurate understanding rather than maximalist inclusivity.

Digital platforms hosting mental health content face particular obligations given their role in propagating diagnostic misinformation. Content claiming that common experiences constitute symptoms of disorders should be flagged or restricted. Algorithms promoting such content because it generates engagement should be modified to prioritize accuracy over virality. Platform policies should distinguish between advocacy and misinformation, supporting the former while limiting the latter.

Research funding priorities must shift toward clarifying diagnostic boundaries and developing better assessment tools. Current instruments like rating scales and structured interviews were validated against populations where clear impairment criteria were enforced. As diagnostic practices drift toward inclusivity, these instruments may no longer reliably distinguish clinical from subclinical presentations. New assessment approaches integrating objective measures of functional capacity, neuropsychological testing, and careful longitudinal evaluation may be necessary to restore diagnostic precision.

The ethical framework guiding these reforms must balance multiple considerations. Autonomy requires respecting individuals' self-understanding and identity claims, but this respect has limits when self-identification undermines systems serving collective interests. Beneficence requires providing support to all who struggle, but this support need not take the form of diagnostic labels that distort medical categories. Justice requires ensuring that those with greatest impairment receive necessary resources, which demands maintaining clear boundaries between pathology and variation. Non-maleficence requires avoiding harm to the severely impaired through resource diversion and trivialization.

Medical professionals possess obligations to maintain diagnostic integrity derived from their role as stewards of medical knowledge and gatekeepers to medical resources. These obligations include applying diagnoses only when criteria are met, resisting pressure to provide diagnoses for validation or accommodation access when impairment is absent, and educating patients about the distinction between diagnosis and identity. Researchers possess obligations to use diagnostic categories rigorously, excluding subclinical presentations from samples meant to study pathology, and developing better methods for distinguishing clinical from normal-range presentations.

Advocates and activists possess obligations to represent their constituencies accurately, neither minimizing the suffering of the severely impaired nor pathologizing common struggles. Social media users possess obligations to share accurate information about medical topics and to avoid claiming diagnoses without proper assessment. Platform developers possess obligations to design algorithms and policies that prioritize accuracy in health information over engagement maximization. Collectively, these obligations constitute an ethical framework for responsible engagement with psychiatric diagnosis.

The restoration of diagnostic clarity will encounter resistance from those who have invested identity and community in expansive diagnostic categories. This resistance is understandable, as asking people to relinquish diagnostic labels they find meaningful appears to invalidate their experiences. However, the validation of experience does not require diagnostic labels. Someone whose struggles with attention are real but subclinical does not need an ADHD diagnosis to have those struggles recognized and addressed. Someone whose sensory sensitivities create genuine challenges does not need an autism diagnosis to warrant accommodation and support. The conflation of validation with diagnosis represents a failure of cultural imagination, a poverty of language that forces all recognition of struggle into medical frameworks.

The philosopher Charles Taylor's concept of the politics of recognition emphasizes that human flourishing requires having one's identity and experiences acknowledged by others. However, Taylor specifies that recognition must be authentic rather than distorted. The authentic recognition of someone experiencing subclinical attentional difficulties acknowledges that their struggles are real while also acknowledging that these struggles fall within normal human variation and do not constitute pathology. Distorted recognition applies a diagnostic label that misrepresents the nature and severity of their difficulties, providing validation through false categorization.

The way forward demands conceptual honesty: applying diagnostic categories according to validated criteria, maintaining functional impairment as the threshold for diagnosis, developing rich non-pathological vocabulary for human variation, and ensuring that validation and support flow through multiple channels rather than being monopolized by medical diagnosis. This approach honors both scientific integrity and human need for recognition, rejecting the false dichotomy that forces us to choose between the two.

The stakes extend beyond abstract debates about diagnostic criteria. Real people with severe impairments depend on diagnostic systems functioning properly to access treatment and accommodation that makes the difference between catastrophic dysfunction and manageable challenge. When those systems degrade through conceptual corruption, these individuals pay the price in denied accommodations, delayed treatment, and trivialized suffering. The restoration of diagnostic precision is not merely a technical matter for specialists but a moral imperative affecting the most vulnerable members of society. We owe them conceptual honesty, which means using diagnostic language accurately, maintaining clear boundaries between pathology and variation, and preserving the tools they need to describe and remediate genuine suffering.

www.ingramcontent.com/pod-product-compliance
Lightning Source LLC
LaVergne TN
LVHW022101200926
848481LV00003B/1016
*9798232225681*